CALL TO WITNESS

(handwritten inscription) Dear Daisy — Thank you for all of your support. *(signature)* 2017

CALL TO WITNESS

One Woman's Battle with Disability, Discrimination and a Pharmaceutical Powerhouse

(handwritten inscription) Daisy — you are beautiful & I can't wait to spend time with you — Cheryl Blackman

By Sherry Blackman

BROAD STREET PUBLISHING OF MONROE COUNTY
East Stroudsburg, PA

Broad Street Publishing of Monroe County
113 West Broad Street
East Stroudsburg, PA 18301

Website: calltowitness.com

First Edition: April 2013
Second Printing: June 2013

Library of Congress Cataloging-in-Publication Data
Blackman, Sherry
    Call to Witness: One Woman's Battle with Disability, Discrimination and a Pharmaceutical Powerhouse / Sherry Blackman—1st ed.

ISBN 978-0-9858229-0-3
    1. Blackman, Sherry   2. Authors, American—21st century—memoir
3. Disability—Discrimination—Pennsylvania—Memoir—Pharmaceutical—
Vaccines—Lawsuit

Cover photo by Stella Alesi © 2013 Stella Alesi.

All material used from *The Spirit of Swiftwater: 100 Years at The Pocono Labs* (Scranton: Scranton University Press, 1998) by Jeff Widmer is used with permission from Scranton University Press.

Typeset, printed and bound in the United States by G&H Soho, Inc. www.ghsoho.com.

Dedication

Sherry dedicates this book to
Erin, Lindsay, Alex, Dakotah and Harley

Jane to her Aunt Mary and Uncle Chauncy,
who built the brick house for her family
that the big bad wolf could never blow down.

Patrick to his parents, Joe and Betty Reilly,
who gave him opportunities,
to his children Kristin, Kyle and Naomi, who inspire him
and to his wife, Malka, who completes him.

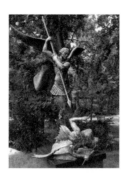

ABOUT THE COVER

St. Michael and Lucifer, the name of the sculpture on the front cover, was photographed at The Umlauf Sculpture Garden & Museum, a non-profit organization founded around the work of American sculptor Charles Umlauf, in Austin, Texas. The sculpture depicts Umlauf's vision of good triumphing over evil, of justice prevailing. Umlauf purposely gave Lucifer, or Evil, a young, attractive face to show the school children how appealing evil can be.

Umlauf Sculpture Garden & Museum is dedicated to providing educational experiences that encourage the understanding and appreciation of sculpture. The accessible sculptures are coated in wax so that anyone with any disability might be able to "see" them with their hands, if need be.

The author would like to thank the staff of Umlauf for their willingness to have one of their sculptures featured on the cover of this book and their excitement to be recognized for their mission for all, regardless of disability, to enjoy the power of Umlauf's work.

Acknowledgements

The author, Sherry Blackman, would like to acknowledge and thank James Rawlins for helping to edit the book—your encouragement has lifted me up more than once during the long writing process. Also, agent Rebecca Pratt, who worked hard and diligently on this project, and whose expertise helped to shape the story. My children Erin, Lindsay and Alex, and grandchildren, Dakotah and Harley, who hold me to life. Jane and Pat, thank you for sharing this story the world needs to hear, and Jane, for all those long afternoon feasts. Lastly, I would like to acknowledge the Presbyterian Church USA for standing up and standing by the marginalized of our society, for risking being controversial, for willing to get the grime of the world under their fingernails, without apology.

Jane Gagliardo would like to acknowledge Toni DeMaio—I love you like a sister. Thank you for bringing Sherry and me together. And Patrick Reilly, who always has my back. As well, I would like to acknowledge my family whom loves me unconditionally (sometimes). Sherry, thank you for taking the story of my life and putting it into words from the heart. You told my story so beautifully. You made it come alive once again. Your words and writing are a gift from heaven.

Also, I would like to acknowledge my grandchildren, John, Nick, Franky, Francesca, the Little Miracle, who have taught me a kind of love that I never knew existed. Even after death love goes on. And my children, Joe, Melanie, Johnny, Jenn, Anthony and June, who gave me the greatest gift, their children and their love. John, you are the love of my life. I've known you more than half my life and loved you just as long. Together we changed the cycle of abuse in our lives, and we made a safe and loving home for our children, and any one else who needed refuge.

Lastly, I would like to acknowledge everyone who thinks that they are throwaways because they have a disability—may you be empowered by my story.

Patrick Reilly would like to acknowledge the great team at Gross McGinley, LLP, whose support, hard work and commitment ensured our success, particularly Allen, Kristin and, Sally.

List of Chapters

—⁓—

CALL TO WITNESS

Prologue

Five stairs. Jane counted them as she leaned on her cane and grabbed the cool railing, dragging her deadened right leg up, one step at a time. It was the final climb into uncertainty. She glanced up at the windows of the Ronald Reagan Federal Building that mirrored a sapphire September sky and the wide Susquehanna River. Everything at that moment, the sky, the water, herself, seemed to drain into some distant, unknowable sea. The air so still, so saturated with the scent of the river, she felt its weight against her, as if she were drowning.

The monolith marble and glass front of the courthouse in Harrisburg, Pennsylvania seemed impermeable. The trial would last for days, her lawyer, Patrick Reilly, warned her. Days—after years of struggling through humiliation, financial difficulties, and the marital strain her lawsuit caused. Would it be worth it, in the end? Would her sense of self be redeemed or be further crushed? Would there be justice for her, and for those who had suffered, and who would suffer, as she had?

Who was she, anyway? A nobody. Someone without power or influence who challenged a pharmaceutical giant, a company whose vaccines coursed through her body, and the bodies of millions of Americans. Who did she think she was?

"Are you ready for the biggest day of your life?" Patrick asked, briefcase in hand, law books tucked under his arm. His thin smile belied his own anxiety she was sure.

There was no turning back now. Behind her, the world. Alongside her, her husband and her lawyer. In front of her, the call to witness.

CHAPTER ONE

"Dead by Morning"

———ᘯᘯ———

Jane woke up. Her body felt as if she had vacated it during the night where remembered dreams seemed to foretell the future. She watched her hand lift the blanket and push it away, but felt nothing—not the soft weave, or her own heat, or the strain of muscle. It was as if she existed outside her own skin and glimpsed herself from afar.

"John, John," she called her husband, but she heard the shower running and he couldn't hear her. She waited, placed her feet on the floor but couldn't sense the carpet beneath them. "Hurry, John," she whispered.

John came into the bedroom, a towel wrapped around his waist, water dripping from his hair. "What's the matter. You look like you've seen a ghost."

"I can't feel my body."

"You know I'd be happy to feel it for you."

She said nothing.

"What do ya mean?"

"I can't feel anything. My feet, my hands, my legs, my arms—they're numb." She started to cry.

John walked to her side and touched her legs. "Can you feel my hands?"

"I can't, John. I can't feel you."

"Check yourself. Maybe you got bit by a spider or something when we were moving all the stuff from the kitchen yesterday."

Jane scrutinized her arms and legs, reached up to search her neck. "I don't see anything; do you see anything on my neck?"

"No nothing. Don't panic. We'll figure this out. I'll call the doctor." But his face said something else, as if he was speaking more to himself than to her.

"Don't leave me, John. Help me into the bathroom. Maybe I'm just tired. Maybe I'll feel better once I take a shower."

"Sure, Babe."

She watched as his hands came beneath her arms and hoisted her up. She couldn't sense his hands. *God, no. . . .* She has to feel his hands. He supported her as she stood and inched forward, dragging her feet toward the bathroom only a few feet away. She rested on the toilet seat. He pulled her nightgown up and off, let it fall to the floor, then turned on the shower.

"I'm going to stay here while you take a shower, ok?" He helped her as she stepped up and into the tub. "If you need help, I'm here. Is this what happens when a woman turns thirty?"

She tried to laugh; she always tried to laugh.

The hot water sprayed down upon her. She knew it was hot because it was steaming; it was the only way she knew. She opened her mouth and swallowed, praying she would feel on the inside of her body what she couldn't feel on the outside. The water washed her tears over her body, leaving no salty trace behind. *Something is wrong, dead wrong.* She studied the water as it cascaded down her chest, over her belly, testing to see if it slid over a nerve anywhere. She touched her body, remembering how her three sons came from that underground part of her. Every nerve in her body had run and hidden in that secret place that she couldn't find, or open the door to.

"How ya doing, Babe?"

"I can't feel the water, John. I can't feel it."

"As soon as you get out, I'll call the doctor. It's probably just a pinched nerve, or nerves. Damn, you worked hard yesterday; it's probably just that."

She didn't answer. *How could every nerve in her body be pinched?*

He dried her off, the same way he once dried off their sons when they were babies, patting them, afraid to rub their skin too hard, and then helped her dress into a loose top and jeans. After throwing on the same jeans he wore yesterday and a fresh tee shirt, he kissed her as she waited on the edge of the bed.

"Can you feel that at least?"

She shook her head.

He walked down the stairs in front of her, so that if she lost her balance, she would fall into him. Her steps were heavy, exaggerated. He cleaned off a chair in the dining room for her to sit on.

"Hey, there isn't too much that a strong cup of coffee won't help cure."

She listened. He wasn't making coffee, but dialed the phone. She focused on a cardinal outside the window, perched inside a forsythia bush, looking like a scarlet heart in a tangled yellow rib cage. It stared back at her, no song rising in its throat. She wondered about her dream she had earlier, a memory really, that replayed itself over and over, when she and her brother were tap dancing on a float in a parade in Warren, Ohio, and all that transpired after. Why had she dreamt about it this morning, on the day she turned thirty? It was a memory, a dream, a nightmare.

John left a message with the answering service, insisting on talking to the doctor right away. His gentle voice tensed as he told the person on the other end of the line of Jane's symptoms, then he hung up. The coffee finished brewing and he served her a cup along with a slice of toast spread with a slab of butter.

She knew he was stalling—he never could straighten out the worry lines of his forehead. He had always been a terrible actor.

After a few minutes, the phone rang.

"The doctor wants to see you right away."

"Listen, you have to be here for the floor guys. I'll drive myself," she said.

He paced over the water-stained plywood. "I can't let you do that—what if, I mean—how can you drive?"

"I don't have sensation in my hands and feet, but I can feel my weight. I can read the speedometer. I made it down the stairs. Maybe I herniated a disk or something. Maybe the feeling will come back in a little bit. Besides, the doctor's only a few blocks away."

"I'll wake Joseph up to go with you."

Joseph, now twelve, their firstborn, was born when she was only eighteen-years-old. She and John had intentionally gotten pregnant so they could be together and escape their abusive households. Her mother didn't talk to her for most of her pregnancy. It was almost as if God had a sense of humor when Joseph was born on her mother's birthday, December 29.

John lumbered up the stairs, shook Joseph awake. She heard their voices like distant music. Johnny, eight-years-old, slept alongside his five-year-old brother, Anthony. Jane imagined feeling the lightness of them in her arms, as she did every night when they were babies, cradling them with late night prayers.

She turned toward the window again; the cardinal flew away.

"Happy birthday, Ma," her son said, rubbing sleep from his eyes.

Like a pilot that uses instruments to fly by, Jane used the car's instruments to drive into Stroudsburg. The landscape seemed remote as she wandered through the one-time mining town in Eastern Pennsylvania, a few miles from the Delaware River. Stroudsburg rested at the edge of black stone mountains, waiting still, it seemed, for its miners to come home. The residue of its coal days was evident in the dust that laced aged buildings high up, as if the city itself suffered from Black Lung.

Elderly men, who were once breaker boys that bloodied their fingers picking out bits of rock from the crushed coal, walked around scarred and arthritic. She thought of old-man hands, dangling at their sides, and contrasted them to the pudgy, dimpled hands of her sons. Nothing held her to life like her boys' hands.

Beneath the road were veins of anthracite. Bits of coal from the breaker had polluted the local waters with toxic run-off. *Maybe she had ingested too many toxins from these old waters. Maybe her body was suffering a cave-in. How much air did she have left?* She thought, there are different kinds of pain—the kind she begged her body to feel now, and the kind she couldn't help feel.

She smelled her father's pipe-fitting hands as if they are near. . . .

They drove down neighborhoods. Houses were aligned close together, most with miniature front yards, ribboned by sidewalks; backyards were bordered with fences. Spring was colliding with winter; breathed warmth on the cold earth. Its breath rose in clouds off the streets and ground.

Maybe there was something else in the air? Jonas Salk made desperate attempts to create a vaccine against the poliovirus—a virus that struck fast and crippled its victims for life, not far from where she lives, in the 1950's.

Her foot pressed on the gas pedal. She watched the speedometer needle move upward, then glanced again at her son. Prayed, *Oh God, please let me be okay.*

At the doctor's office, a nurse ushered Jane into an examining room after a fifteen-minute wait. Joseph stayed behind, looking paralyzed in the chair.

"So what's going on, Jane? John called and said you were having a hard time this morning. He seemed quite alarmed."

"I can't feel my body—even though John is more than happy to compensate." She forced a laugh.

"Let's take a look and see what's going on."

Dr. Lesser shined a tiny flashlight into her eyes, lifted and dropped her limbs, checked her heart, blood pressure, reflexes.

"Still no sensation?" he asked.

"No. What's going on with me? Is it because I strained myself yesterday? I've strained myself before, but not like this."

"I want you to go to a neurologist right away. I will make a call to Dr. Barclay. He's near the hospital."

"What do you think is wrong?"

"I don't know, Jane. But I suspect he will. Don't wait. I know you, Jane. You're a tough, strong-headed woman. Don't wait to go."

She stumbled as she climbed off the exam table.

When Joseph saw her, he rushed to take his mother's arm.

"Dr. Barclay will see you right away," the receptionist said.

They drove a few blocks away to the neurologist's office near Pocono Medical Center, the community hospital.

"What's a neurologist?" Joseph asked.

"Where you go when you are nervous, I think," she said, trying to disarm the bomb that was already exploding inside her.

"Are you nervous, Mom?"

"Yea, Joseph, I am."

The waiting room was busy. They waited a long time. Jane wondered what the receptionist at Dr. Lesser's office meant when she said that Dr. Barclay would see them right away.

"What do you think, Joseph, we'll go home to a new kitchen floor?"

Jane imagined her food and her tenant's food spoiling out on the back stoop—meat thawing, dripping down and staining the cement landing, cold eggs warming, milk turning sour. How would she manage to help John move everything back into the kitchen?

An hour passed. Joseph was antsy, looking at a car magazine.

Dr. Barclay appeared in the hallway and escorted Jane to an examining room. Being short, she had to wiggle onto the table as the thin paper crackled beneath her. The room smelled aseptic, with a tinge of sickness. He broke a Q-tip in half and poked her body—her neck, back—places she couldn't see.

No sensation.

"Get dressed, and I will be back in a couple of minutes." When he returned twenty minutes later he said, "I suspect you have Multiple Sclerosis. You need to go to the hospital right away and be started on steroid IV therapy. If you don't get there by tonight, you'll probably be dead in the morning. If it isn't MS, it's probably Lou Gehrig's Disease."

"What the hell are you talking about?"

"Multiple Sclerosis—a disease where the body's own defense system attacks myelin, the fatty substance that surrounds and protects the nerve fibers in the central nervous system."

"So let me get this right. You poke me with a *fuckin'* Q-tip a dozen times over my body and you make this sweeping diagnosis? If I don't go to the hospital right now, I'll be dead?"

"This is the only disease that presents itself this way," he said, with no inflection change in his voice.

"I'm not going to the hospital without more information," she said, her voice cracking. "I need to talk to my husband."

"I won't be responsible for the outcome if you don't get to the hospital right away. Do you understand?"

She remembered her mother swimming in a sea of white hospital sheets, her body broken and bleeding like a false Christ that couldn't die or be resurrected under her father's fists, and her mouth frothing from too many tranquilizers. Hospitals were where the powerless go.

"You're an asshole, you know that?" She stormed out of his office.

"What's the matter, Mom?" Joseph asked when she emerged from the hallway.

"Don't worry; the doctor's an asshole. He doesn't know shit."

At home, John opened the backdoor where he had been waiting. She just wanted to go inside their home, hear her two younger sons' voices even if they were fighting; she wanted to smell the new vinyl floors. She wanted to fall into John's arms to keep from falling apart.

She struggled up the few backdoor steps, "What did the doctor say?"

Jane waited until Joseph disappeared down the short hallway, through the kitchen, into the living room.

"He says he thinks I have Multiple Sclerosis, tells me, if I don't go to the hospital now, I could be dead by morning."

She saw his face sink into itself; the darkness of his eyes flashed then faded. His skin turned ashen. He pulled her close and held her. He said nothing, but pressed to his chest she heard his wild heart.

"The floor guys never showed up either."

"So, let me get this right. Not only am I going to be dead by morning, I'll never be able to see my new kitchen floor?"

They laughed, trying to push away the sorrow that wound itself around them like the serpent on the Staff of Asclepius.

CHAPTER TWO

Rerun of an Ancient Broadcast

Jane lay on her bed that night and remembered what she could never forget.

Memorial Day, 1960, in Warren, Ohio. All the folks flood High Street. Dozens of men carry a giant American flag among them like a sheet held out to catch falling stars, stretching over the entire street as they pass the courthouse. The flag billows as if trying to throw the stars back into the sky.

The float drifts through the parade. Jane spanks the hardwood with her tap shoes, listens to the rhythmic clack, and then brushes her heel right. Her entire child body is a percussive instrument—as if her tiny heart produced a sound the entire world could hear. Her older brother, Dominic, dances alongside. They are wearing matching outfits, tan bolero jackets with white tailored shirts beneath, wide pants, their shoes a black patent leather that catches the light and dark shadows of their movements.

The truck pulls them forward. Television cameras focus on her buoyant body. The metal plates on her soles alone weigh her down to earth. Then the truck slows, lurches forward, throwing her off balance. She catches herself, clutches her brother's arm in such a way that it seems a part of the dance. It was as if she was always catching her brother.

Faces stare at them now; fingers point. She wants to reach back. Women with cotton candy hair smile at them and then clap. She sees her mom, her hand waving more insistently than all the rest, her smile brilliant. Her father stands alongside, his lips crooked and tight as if he is clenching his jaw. She loses the musical beat for a second.

Grilled-sausage smoke creates pillars that hold up nothing. The smell of yeasty pizza dough wafts from the church booth, making the air smell like her mother's hands. Her mother made pizzas and sold them to the church for money to buy the costumes they are wearing. For a moment, the factory air doesn't smolder with burning tires and scorched metal. Helium balloons wave back and forth in clusters, like lifesaver-colored grapes.

Don't let the parade stop. Let it go on and on.

She was seven-years-old then. The ancient broadcast had endless reruns in her head, and maybe now, her body. It was as if she was always trying to find her way back to that moment between moments, when no one could touch her. Then the story was only about her and her brother, who was three years older than she, performing on top of that float.

Back home, after the parade, her father raged at her mother for spending money on their costumes. He grabbed the thin collar of her mother's calico dress between the fingers of his left hand and then slapped her face with his right until her cheeks rushed with blood and her lips bled. Her mother crawled . . . crawled away from his anger, but she knew there was no place to hide. She pleaded for him to stop. Her words were stained red.

Thunderous blows to her mother's skull. His hands reeked of steel, of burning steel.

His hands too calloused to feel her mother's softness or the scars of old beatings that roped her skin in places seen and unseen . . . hands like fire, the color of flame, yet hard as figured stone. He opened them to a map of madness.

"Leave her alone," Jane screamed, feeling as if she was falling head-long off the float onto the hard pavement, with everyone's eyes fastened on the next float, the other performance. She was invisible now. She stood barefoot, her tap shoes tucked away in the closet where she had secreted her brother. Her father's metallic sweat sickened her as she stared him in the eye. His fist uncurled like a snake about to strike. He stepped back. She waited. He turned away, smaller than he had ever been before.

Her grit was forged on an anvil of pain watching her mother being abused day after day. She called the ambulance, a number she knew by heart, a number she would never forget.

Wounded, she had always been wounded, even though he didn't hit her. He had written upon her small girl bones a script of violence.

The past is always the present no matter how hard you try to escape it, she thought.

"Well, I didn't die. I'm here, asshole doctor," she mumbled to herself. She had more feeling in her limbs that morning, but there were streaks of burning numbness still. She turned to gaze at the photograph of herself and John on the bedside table. They were a study in contrasts, despite the fact that they both were of Italian descent. His eyes were the color of dark olives, his hair thick and brown. He was six feet, two inches tall and she reached five feet. He stood over and around her, protecting her from the fists of the world.

John too had grown up in a household where his father beat his mother. Italian blood boiled with holy and unholy passion, she knew. Both she and John had decided long ago they would be a refuge of safety for each other and their three children, and whoever needed sanctuary. He had the hands of a kind warrior, solid and strong, that could carry the weight of her entire world in them—all three boys at once.

While he slept, she saw the lines around his eyes had deepened with every mile he drove a truck. He had been transporting hazardous materials. Truckers called them hot loads. He was over the road for two or three nights and sometimes he was home every day, depending on what loads had to be delivered.

He had made her laugh long ago—was it the laugh lines that deepened? His humor caught her like one who is caught in a maelstrom or whirlpool—there was no escaping being swallowed up by it, only to emerge to find that same buoyancy she discovered when she tap danced long ago.

CHAPTER THREE

Connaught Laboratories, Four Years Later, 1987

―――⚬〰⚬―――

The room reeked of burnt coffee inside the Unemployment Office. Dozens of people were applying to work the *flu line* at Connaught. Childbearing women, retired men, and the optimistic young waited, holding individual numbers in their hands. They listened for their number to be called. Numbers erased identity, Jane thought, making people easier to reject and ignore.

Vertically challenged, a little stocky, with medium length dark brown hair, what distinguished her from the crowd, other than her distinct Italian heritage? She clutched her thin resume—grateful just to feel the stiff white paper between her fingers.

In that dull space, she remembered her birthday four years earlier. Something had died that day—the feeling that all would be well, that she had some control over the future. Fear had wound its way around her, sometimes tightening, until she struggled to breathe. She wondered often what roused the numbing snake that slept coiled inside her, awakening at different moments.

The diagnosis of Multiple Sclerosis hadn't yet been confirmed— leaving it unnamed, disempowered it in some way. Yet she wondered if the doctor had been right. Too often she couldn't feel her own skin. Sometimes there was a tingling that ran up and down her spine and legs that seemed to stop at her ankles.

At thirty-four, she was a few pounds overweight. Her breasts were heavy and large. She once nursed each one of her sons. Now in their teens, they were still sucking the life out of her it seemed.

Everyone in the Stroudsburg area wanted to work the flu line—it was a way to get one's foot in the door of the only corporate giant in the region. Those who were hired would assist the young and the old in obtaining the flu vaccine.

A small woman with dark, medium length, silver-streaked hair and hazel eyes came into the room and called Jane's number. She introduced herself as Madeline, a Personnel Representative for Connaught. Madeline carried herself with professional grace in her gray, man-tailored suit with the oversized shoulder pads. Her voice was pleasant, her speech as fluid as water.

Within minutes, Jane learned Madeline was Italian, divorced, and the mother of sons, and was self-supporting. They found themselves sharing the common ground of maternal concerns. But then the conversation shifted. Madeline talked of Connaught as if the company was a person, a parent, and employees were grafted into the family tree with roots that ran so deep in this Pennsylvania soil that it anchored the entire region from eroding into oblivion and poverty.

Jane mustered up the courage to slip Madeline her resume. *Maybe Connaught could be the "parent" she never had.*

"Ninety-nine percent of the people who apply for flu line jobs don't even know what a resume is."

"I want to work for Connaught," Jane said. "I need a good, secure job, and I will take any position you can offer. My husband and I promised our sons we would send them to college. I'm a good worker."

"We have a new Customer Service Department that just started a year ago. I think you'll be perfect for it. It's headed up by two nurses, and they're looking to increase the head count. I'll pass on your resume to the person responsible for hiring in that department. Just be patient; give it about a week."

Jane called twice a week over the next month until she was promised an interview with Connaught. After consulting women's magazines, she bought a new suit from *Fashion Bug*—tan with a light blue camisole underneath, a pair of brown heels and a purse to match.

A few days before, she received a packet of material she had requested about the company, following the advice of women's magazines. She studied it, memorized details about the company's mission statement and its history. The company was the producer of the first Salk polio vaccine which brought an end to the polio epidemic in the 1950's. Connaught had become the world leader in producing immunizations and serums against diphtheria, smallpox, tetanus, meningitis, rabies, and influenza.

Reading Connaught's history made her shiver, conjuring up images of her childhood vaccinations all over again. Steel syringes, the sterilizing autoclave open, revealing more nightmare-producing syringes. She had the small globe-like scar of the vaccine boaster near her left shoulder.

Jonas Salk was hailed as a miracle worker. He refused to patent the vaccine as he desired only to eradicate the crippling disease that stole childhoods, paralyzed limbs, and made *iron lungs* a household word.

Swiftwater, Pennsylvania—who knew the small town was such a landmark on the map of humanity? The more she read, the hungrier she was to secure a job at Connaught and make her own mark . . . the thought exhilarated her. The company had it all—good benefits and good pay, tuition reimbursement, if she decided to go to college. Somehow she had to sell herself as never before. Maybe one day the company would find a vaccine to prevent such diseases as Multiple Sclerosis.

She said nothing to her tenant, Judy, who already worked in Connaught's legal department as a paralegal. She wouldn't either, until she landed the job.

The interview was scheduled on a Wednesday. She would prepare the weekly pot of spaghetti sauce early, let it simmer all day until the entire house swelled with the fragrance of plum tomatoes, garlic, oregano and basil, a plucked garden crushed and meshed. Washing and dicing the tomatoes, sautéing them in the pot, watching them soften and bleed and break down into each other reminded her of family. She lamented the fact that she didn't like Italian food . . . but it didn't matter, her family did, and John expected it every Wednesday and Sunday, like a sacramental meal. It had become a tradition she never broke, even when he was on the road, away from home. Somehow when she cooked spaghetti, he felt miles closer than he really was.

Before she walked out the door she read through her notes once more, committing what she could to memory. She sprayed a bit more hairspray to tame her wavy hair, layered so it wasn't too bushy, and then dabbed Jessica McClintock cologne on to mask the spaghetti sauce aroma that was trapped in the weave of her polyester suit.

Connaught security guards wouldn't let her beyond the gate without a pass.

"You need to go to Building 37, where the flu is made. Just head for the stack where the smoke is spewing from."

She saw the white smoke and followed it, parking in the Visitors Parking Lot.

"You better get this job," she argued with herself. "You didn't pay a three-year subscription to that women's magazine for nothing."

Jane walked by the old horse stalls where Pasteur, Merieux, Fitzgerald, Salk—the hero-scientists—stabled their horses for their medical experiments decades earlier. Other buildings, low and small in comparison to the factory that dominated the landscape, looked like barns for animals, maybe for the monkeys Salk used for his first clinical trials for the polio vaccine. A pond, not far away, shimmered with an oily sheen.

She opened the door to Building 37 just as the wind changed direction and blew against it. A strong odor, one she couldn't identify, assaulted her as she entered—something like rubbing alcohol and pine cleaner mixed together.

A woman down the hallway, sitting at a desk, looked up at Jane.

"I'm here for an interview with Alice Wilson and John McCoy," Jane said.

"They are expecting you." The name plate on the woman's desk said Linda Possinger, a tall woman who would turn both men's and women's heads alike for different reasons. Men, for lust; women, for jealousy. She was a well-dressed, long-legged blond in a black suit. Guess she read the same women's magazines, Jane surmised and smirked, following her to an office off to the left. No one else was there in the area waiting, unlike at the Unemployment Office. *A good sign.*

"Can I get you a drink?" the bombshell offered.

"No, thank you," *but a gin and tonic would go real well right about now to calm my nerves*, she wanted to say. It was as if the woman read her mind and smiled. No one was in the office, so she waited, trying to recall every word she had read about the company—damn, she couldn't recall a blasted thing.

Alice Wilson, the head of Customer Service, RN after her name, entered the office. She was the opposite of Linda—bare-faced, no make-up to warm her sallow-toned skin. She wore her mousy blond hair straight and nondescript. A plain blue shirt hung loose over a pair of corduroy pants.

Alice extended her non-manicured hand and offered a limp handshake.

"Look, let's get to the point. I need people who are positive, who are team players, people who will make the company a priority in their lives. You will create the first impression of who the company is as soon as you open your mouth on the other end of a phone call. They won't know, nor will they care if you are beautiful or ugly, if you are well-dressed or sloppy. They are calling for information and you need to be on it, do you understand? When you say, 'Connaught Laboratories, how may I help you,' your voice and manner better be sincere, confident and convincing. You are expected to defend the company no matter what your personal beliefs are on childhood vaccines. And, oh by the way, were your children vaccinated?"

Her barrage caused Jane to gasp for air. She cleared the back of her throat. "Of course my children were vaccinated." *She wanted to add, what, you don't think I am a good mother? Why wasn't there an article about childhood vaccines in the women's magazines anyway? Must have missed that issue.*

"You'll be taking orders from all over the country, do you understand, from every corner of every state, from people who talk like you and people who don't. You'll be speaking with doctors and nurses, pharmacists and our own sales reps. No matter why they are calling, you must act as if you have everything under control, that there is no problem in handling whatever issue they have."

"I understand." Alice had no idea who Jane was, how she had grown up with three brothers, how she was never allowed to cry, no matter what happened.

The door behind her opened and a man of average height and medium build, with red hair and blue eyes, disheveled, with a crooked tie, joined them. He extended his hand before Jane even had a chance to stand up.

"John McCoy. I'm sorry for being late. I have two daughters, and they are keeping me so busy I can't even get out of the house dressed straight." His eyes were as transparent as he seemed.

Alice disengaged . . . children were not of interest, at least it appeared that way. McCoy ignored Alice and began to tell the story of how he came to Connaught only a few months ago. "I wanted to live in the mountains," he said. "You know, clean air and all that."

Outside the smoke swirled and curled with a sudden downwind.

"We just moved down the road, on the lake, in a new development. Best move I ever made."

They spoke for a long time. Alice was silent when McCoy said, "I think you are exactly what we are looking for. When would you be able to start if you were offered the job?" He looked toward Alice, who looked as if she was sucking on a sourball. "Alice, do you have any more questions?"

"What was the last book you read?"

"*Green Eggs and Ham*, by Dr. Seuss," Jane said.

McCoy laughed, thank God.

Alice's lips grew thin and flat. "We'll let you know," she blurted out.

McCoy walked Jane to the door. He whispered, "Don't mind Alice; she's not a people person. You'll be hearing from me."

Outside, the air smelled of burning eggs.

Three weeks later, McCoy called Jane, offering her ten dollars an hour to start, with benefits and retirement. Jane wanted to wake her husband up from sleep—but he had to make a run that night to Consolidated Freight Ways Terminal in Akron, Ohio. She decided instead to tell Judy, their tenant, and rushed next door.

"Connaught is hiring anyone these days," Judy said.

"It's a new department. I'll be great at this job." Jane stood for a short while in Judy's kitchen, looking at the kitchen floor that was now four years old, the same she had installed in her own kitchen. She scuffed her feet. Shouldn't have bothered to tell her; she's not happy about it. "I'll talk to you later, Judy, when you're feeling more hostile, I mean hospitable." She shut the door with more force than necessary.

The kids were still at school. Jane sauntered upstairs and slipped into bed with John. "I got the job, ten dollars an hour, with benefits and retirement. Do you believe it?"

He was on his side, facing her. The early afternoon sun peeked under the shade looking like the background of an icon, gold paint illuminating something divine between the vinyl slots. His right arm reached for her and drew her near. She inhaled the musk of his skin, the faint dust of diesel fumes that lingered somewhere on him, his breath maybe. His hair was mussed, sticking out in different directions. The warmth of him seduced her to dream, and she did for a moment about what life will be like at Connaught. She would finally be able to help lift the family out of debt and give them a sense of security they had never had.

"I got it. Do you believe it? I got the job."

"I'm proud of you, Babe, real proud of you." His hand caressed her arm and scooped her breast almost as if drawn to it by a magnet. His hand was so large that it measured half way across her belly.

She unbuttoned her shirt, unhooked her bra and pressed herself against him. This familiarity, this yearning, healed her in some invisible place—flesh against flesh, the heat, the pressure of his hand at her back, the cave their bodies made under the blankets, the darkness that felt more like light. She yanked off her pants and left them encircling her feet until she kicked them down deeper into the dark. She couldn't feel the soles of her feet, or her toes, so she used the side of her leg to free her of the entanglement. This was the way they always celebrated good news.

His hand traveled her belly, her upper leg, her thigh, cutting her almost, as if a loving scalpel, opening her up, exposing bone and muscle. There was no gravity between them. He moved off his side and she moved her body beneath him, and they laughed at the awkwardness of their bodies even now, so many years later, as they did that first night when they were seventeen.

Her body ached for him then and it ached for him now. Her hands traced the notches of his backbone, the mass of his back, touching the patches of hair that were never there before—a sign of age, a warning of time. She tried to memorize him. Her hands, what if they stopped feeling again, what if her nerve endings unraveled and died if she really had MS?

March 12th marked the beginning of her new life. The day was warmer than the past few, the air hinting of spring, the light stretching a bit longer every day. Driving to Connaught for her first day of her first ever career, she believed all would be different now. Life was good—her boys were doing well at school, John was president of the East Stroudsburg Youth Association, she was helping to sell tickets for the church bazaar, and there were the football games where all the teams' moms worked on organizing events and selling refreshments. Her dream complete now, if only the job worked out.

At the security gate, the guard instructed her on where to go to obtain a badge and a parking tag. Inside the security office she watched a video on security and safety. Building 37—where the flu vaccine was made, the guard told her to go. Walking toward the building, she noticed the smoke was heavy in the stagnant air and left a film on her skin. She reached for the door that had the same dew-like substance on it, wiped her hand on her scarf, and then checked to see if there was any stain.

That same smell of alcohol and pine cleaner hit her again upon entry, as did the rank-smelling smoke choking the air outside. Rose Kindrew met her at the entrance, as if she had been alerted to her coming. Rose's long, coffee-colored hair was loose and straight. Her voice had a lilt of laughter even as she showed Jane around. Standing close to her, Jane smelled the smoke on Rose's clothes amid the sterile pine and alcohol odors. Like Alice, she wore no make-up, a pair of jeans and a tee-shirt.

Minutes later, Alice called Jane into her office. "I really hope that if this job isn't for you, you will have the decency to come and tell me."

"Of course, Alice. Of course, I will." *Fuck you. You may be an intelligent bully, but I've stood up to my bullies before. You won't be the first, and I doubt you will be the last.*

Dismissed by a nod of the head, Jane entered an office and counted six small cubicles butted up against a wall. The room, a light shade of gray, was no larger than her kitchen back at the duplex. But there were no windows to view the corporate campus, no fresh air. Maybe that's the point—there was no fresh air to inhale. Outside the air was nothing more than the residue of whatever brewed in the labs. The scent of the women mixed together in the enclosed space. Phones rang like alarm clocks.

"You'll be working both shifts—the second one ends at eight in the evening. We have to do this to accommodate the West Coast," Rose said. "I'll put you on alternate days so that you can get a handle on both shifts. Here's a list of the products you need to know about inside and out."

Names bounced back and forth inside her skull like ping-pong balls and it took everything in her mind to swat them back and commit them to memory. Her brain tissue seemed little more than white soggy paper that housed scribbles—pharmaceutical names, so many syllables, so much chemistry compressed into letters, names without faces or colors or stories, at least not yet. Tripedia and Daptacel, otherwise known as DTaP; JE-Vax, otherwise known as the Japanese Encephalitis vaccine; Tdap or Adacel; Typhim Vi against Typhoid. . . .

A whole new language, a new way of speaking, words that saved lives, Jane mused as she swore at them to stay put inside her. Did they have a vaccine against fear or falling down the first day on the job? She read through the product information on diphtheria, tetanus, and pertussis vaccines.

She read through Centers for Disease Control (CDC) documents until she was dizzy. . . . Formaldehyde, used as an antimicrobial preservative, mouse brain used as a culture for Japanese Encephalitis, Thimerosal, Chick embryo fibroblast tissue culture, monkey kidney tissue culture for DTaP and Polio. . . .

A vocabulary of disease and cure . . . she imagined Dr. Salk growing cultures on monkey kidneys in the small barns she passed before entering Building 37. So much sacrifice for humans. Did they have any-thing to do now with those two words that wrote themselves at the end of day across her body, leaving room for little else: *Multiple Sclerosis?* But if she turned a deaf ear, would that beast walk away, find someone else to live in? Erase the words from your mind, she repeated to herself; erase them from your body. *No one, nothing, is going to stand in your way here. You've arrived, and now you must figure out a way to stay.*

CHAPTER FOUR

Life & Death in the Power of a Needle

Amy, a young mother living in Western Pennsylvania, was driving to the grocery store, then to the bank, checking off her to-do list. Her thirteen-month-old son, Chad, played with sounds that flowed and stammered in half-formed words in his mouth as he sat snug and strapped in his car seat.

The sunroof was open. Amy readjusted the mirror to keep one eye on Chad. Outside, the trees were bursting into a firework of lime green, full of luminosity and sparkle. She drove the long way home so he could catch a nap.

Chad cried out. She turned around, expecting him to have awakened with a start. Something black flapped its wings over his face. She screamed. It was a bat, a bat clutching its teeth into his face. She slammed on the brakes and the car lurched to a halt. Chad's shrieking and groaning were muffled by the bat whose teeth and claws were buried in his flesh.

Amy reached back, screaming at the creature; then clutching it with her hand, she crushed its bones between her fingers. She wrestled with the dark angel until its guts spewed out onto her face and arm, until blood spurted out its mouth and over her face. She expected the blood to be black. She saw Chad's blood drip down his face and onto his shirt.

"It's going to be ok, baby; it's going to be ok. Mommy's got it. Don't worry. Mommy won't let anything happen to you," she said in a panicked voice.

She couldn't reach back to comfort him—the bat was in her hand and she had to steer the car. Her fingers kept rolling and crushing the bat's toothpick-like bones until they splintered.

"God have mercy," she prayed.

She sped past her house, driving as fast as her adrenaline-hot legs would drive her.

Amy jolted the car into park outside the Emergency Room door and bolted into the hospital.

"Someone help me. Someone help me." She's held the bat at a distance from her body, looking like a vampire. A nurse ran toward her with a plastic bag and commanded Amy to let go, but Amy's fingers wouldn't open.

"My baby, my baby's in the car. The bat bit him. Help me, please help me." Her words shattered the calm. The bat's limp body fell into the bag.

She raced to the car, the nurse flying behind her, unbuckled the straps on the car seat, and lifted her child to her chest. She couldn't tell whose wild heart it was that beat so fast.

His cries were guttural, ancient, primordial. . . . "Please help us, please help us." She wasn't sure if she was praying to God or to the nurses.

"We need an immediate shipment of the Imovax Rabies Vaccine," the voice said on the other end of phone. "We've got a mother and a toddler who need it STAT."

"We'll get the vaccine out to you immediately. Tell me where it needs to be shipped to," Jane responded.

After the nurse gave Jane all the information, the nurse told Jane what had happened. Jane knew the nurse had to be a mother. *Once a woman gives birth to a child she becomes pregnant with the whole world, forever.* And she knew at the end of the shift, Jane too would have to tell others if for no other reason than to rid herself of the horrific images in her imagination, of black wings covering a baby's face, fangs gripping the cheek just beneath the eyes.

"We should have the vaccine on hand, but we don't. We don't get much of a call for it. It doesn't have a long shelf life, you know?" There's a hint of apology in the nurse's voice.

"Don't worry. I promise it'll be there within hours, even if I have to bring it myself. Your hospital is only a few hours away. Are the mother and child doing okay?"

"I'm not sure the mother will ever be okay again, if you know what I mean. I wouldn't be."

Never open the window, never open the roof, the sky may just cave in.

Within an hour the rabies vaccine was on its way. Jane sat back in her chair. The shift was coming to an end. The others were packing up their things—straightening their desks, order forms, pens, wiping the phone clean with an antiseptic, tossing the dirtied paper cloth into the garbage.

The rabies vaccine would save the woman and child, but it had saved her as well, in a way. *Maybe salvation always came that way—saving both the injured and the healer.* She was no healer, but the company, and she as part of it, had the power to save. No matter what, protect the company Rose had said; Alice had said it too.

Connaught had given her a great gift, something no one ever had given her before—a sense of personal worth apart from all others, a sense of power.

The next morning Jane fried eggs for breakfast for the first time since beginning her job as her stomach lurched at the mere thought since she smelled eggs burning all day.

Her mother called, told her, "Your father told everyone at the American Legion Hall that you're working for Connaught—he's real proud of you."

Jane said nothing at first. The words hung like a noose. Love and hate existed side by side, or maybe they were two parts of the same mystery. Not even violence destroyed love.

Here she was, working at a pharmaceutical company, like the companies that manufactured all the pills her mother ate by the handfuls more than once to escape the love-hate of her marriage. More than once, Jane had come home from high school to find her mother on the floor, foaming at the mouth. Death, better than life for the woman whose heart was so wounded, so bruised, it was better to stop it. She wanted to say, I'm glad Dad is proud of me; I only wish I could say I was ever proud of him.

Those pills were the very reason Jane refused to take medications, no matter what her diagnosis. How many times had she called the ambulance to come and save her mother? How many times had she called the cops, who did nothing back then, considering it a family dispute, and a husband had the right to hit his wife? Not even the hospital rescued her mother, or their family from her father. How many times did a woman have to be admitted? How many bones had to be broken? How many bruises must bloom under her skin before anyone would do anything? Her mother screamed out even when she was silent, protecting the man she married, the man who crept into other women's beds and bodies.

Her father's praise was like prickers to the back of her head. It felt like a goodwill offering, only the words had thorns, thorns that were so embedded inside she thought if maybe this was what caused her limbs and hands to stop feeling sometimes, just as she had stopped feeling for him so long ago.

"Mom, thanks for telling me. It makes me feel good and bad all at the same time, you know? I just want it to feel good."

Her words met with silence and the noose dangled over her head for a few more seconds.

"Your father didn't mean to be so hurtful when you were growing up."

She knew better than to follow those words; she felt the noose around her neck, pulling tighter.

"You may choose to believe that, Mom, but I don't." For a moment, just for a moment, she wanted to be her mother's hero again.

———⟋⟍⟍⟍⟋———

"Good Morning, Connaught Laboratories, how may I help you today?"

No voice, only sobbing greeted Jane on the other end of the line.

"You're a murderer. You killed my baby. I hope you BURN IN HELL!"

"Excuse me?"

"You should never get another good night's sleep again. You murdered my baby."

"You must have the wrong number." Jane felt herself trembling. Murdered a woman's baby?

"Are you the company that makes DTP?" The woman's voice grew in volume and anger.

"Yes."

"Then you murdered my baby."

Linda grabbed the phone from Jane's hand . . . she'd been listening . . . she'd seen the shock on Jane's face. "May I help you?"

A pause, then Linda said, "I will transfer you to the legal department—" the legal department, where her tenant, Judy, worked as a paralegal. Linda placed the receiver down.

"It happens sometimes, Jane. Don't let it shake you. Take a break; get yourself calmed down. Take as much time as you need and then come back."

Jane walked outside—the wind blew the smoke eastward, away from her. Liz, one of the team leaders, was there, sucking on a cigarette, exhaling tobacco smoke into the already tainted air. After she told Liz what had happened, Liz said, "Sometimes it happens. Sometimes babies have adverse reactions. But the vaccines save lives. You need to focus on the gains, not the losses."

As if lives were numbers on the bottom line, and Connaught was God.

"My own children have these vaccines running in their blood. Are they in some kind of danger?"

"If they were, you'd already know about it."

Would she? Were the vaccines she had had as a kid lurking in hidden places inside her that was shearing off the nerve sheath that is Multiple Sclerosis?

Back inside, Jane wended her way to Alice's office. "I need to know more about how vaccines are made."

"You won't understand it. You don't have the education."

"Try me."

Alice was right, Jane didn't understand Connaught's recipe for DPT—detoxified by formaldehyde, thimerosal, aluminum. Words so jumbled together they were knitted into one long strand of chaos. "Cultured . . . harvested . . . added to—" a recipe of metals and toxins and purifying agents.

"Take the material home. If you aren't up to the job, have the decency to give it to someone who is," Alice said.

"I will."

Outside, the smoke burned the air like a perpetual hell.

CHAPTER FIVE

Secrets of the Earth

"Is there some kind of math, you know, divine math, John, where one baby is saved by a rabies vaccine and another is killed by the DPT vaccine?"

"I don't know, Babe. Who can answer that question? You just have to trust that what's meant to be will be. Look, I drive a truck, right? I spew pollutants into the air every day, the same that scientists say are causing global warming, just to bring to the masses a sugary drink that has no redeeming value, and that doctors say leads to diabetes—at least you're in a job that saves lives," John said.

"I know, I know you're right, but sometimes it just gets to me. You've no idea how it felt yesterday when I got that call accusing me of murdering a baby."

"Come here, Babe. I'll make you feel better."

It was early morning, Saturday, a day of reprieve. The boys were asleep in the rooms down the hall. John pulled her toward him.

"Do you really think having sex is going to make anything better?"

"No, but it'll definitely give you something bigger to think about."

"You're an idiot, you know that?"

"Yep, now let me teach you something."

Every time they made love, every time he loomed over her or under her, she felt safer from the violence that raged both inside her and in the world, but this morning something was different—he couldn't help her forget; he couldn't silence the woman's voice.

Sex—it's a pill, of sorts, for whatever ails you, for the disconnect you feel from yourself and another. Jane dressed and headed downstairs to the kitchen to make breakfast. She thought about the woman who had lost her baby. Would she rush into bed to conceive again or would she turn away forever from the child's father? *A mother dies with her child.*

John left for the road. She would do her household things and then take the boys to Connaught and let them fish in the campus pond for a while since it was Saturday. The pond was far enough away from the smoke stacks, and it was a windless day.

Johnny, Anthony and Joseph, all on the brink of puberty and adolescence, packed into the car, reels and tackle boxes in tow, a basket of food for the always-hungry, and a book to read—anything to get her mind off of the last few days' events.

On campus, sandbags were stacked outside the flu vaccine building—building 87. *What the hell, now what?* The air clung to the smell of fire even when the smoke stacks emitted nothing.

At the pond, Jane didn't bother to pull her book out. She sat and watched her sons bait their hooks with worms they had dug up from the yard, cast their lines into the pond that had lost its algae blanket, yet still reflected a fish-like shimmer. They ate bologna and cheese sandwiches, sucked down bottles of *Gatorade*, engaged in a contest of who could chomp the chips the loudest when a spray of sharp crumbs landed on the water.

A few hours later, after catching a few largemouth bass and sunfish, Joseph punctured a large stringer hook through the fishes' mouths and Anthony and Johnny fought for the privilege of carrying them to the car —the three of them damp with sweat and pond water, stained with fish blood, yet they wore the grin of victory. They'd clean them at home, on the back stoop, flicking eyeballs at one another, skimming fish scales that would fly onto their arms and cling like slimy suns.

On Monday, Alice called Jane into the office and handed her two letters, one from upper management, another from a client, expressing kudos for jobs well done. She didn't appear happy about giving them to Jane. She then offered her a copy of each, slipping them into her file.

"Thought you would like to see these," she said.

"Yes, thanks." Jane unfolded the letters.

After reading them, she looked up at Alice and wondered if the reason Alice had moved up the corporate ladder was due to her no nonsense personality. It was the late eighties, the decade of women emerging onto the corporate scene, but not often treated as an equal. Women wore men's suits to work, even ties. It seemed this woman had no room for reproduction in her life, only production.

"Oh, and here's a memo that just came across my desk," she added.

Jane read it—"Don't eat the fish out of the pond." No explanation. "What the hell is this?"

"I don't know. Something must have happened over the weekend." "But my kids—"

"What about your kids?" Alice looked up, her mouth downturned, saying more than her words.

"Nothing."

That afternoon, she and a co-worker, Kathleen, a smart, beautiful, and witty woman, walked over to the Swiftwater Inn, across the street from the campus. The white clapboard and green-shuttered inn with a two-storied porch had once been a stagecoach stop where travelers refreshed themselves with a bit of libation while dusting themselves off. Now, it was an icon.

Inside, she read about the Inn's history on the back of the menu before ordering:

> In the 1890s, a Brooklyn man suffering from cholera came to the Poconos and bedded down at the Swiftwater Inn to recover. There he met, fell in love with and married the innkeeper's daughter.
>
> He married well. His wife had inherited a large sum of money and some land across from the inn. The man, a physician, recovered. As a bacteriologist, he used the land to open a lab, Pocono Biological Laboratories. That company formed the

basis of one of the world's leading suppliers of drugs and vaccines . . . an economic powerhouse in Monroe County.

"Did you ever read this?" Jane asked Kathleen.

"Not really. Who cares how this place came to be? The only thing that matters is that it's within walking distance of work, a quick fix for the thirsty. I do remember hearing about a group that called themselves the Swiftwater Monks—think I'll reestablish the group, starting right now." Kathleen ordered a liquid appetizer.

"I heard about them—they used to dress in robes like real monks and had titles—Scribe Monk, Nectar Monk, right?"

"Yea . . . hmmm . . . think I'll call myself Relations Monk. It's just one of those days."

"Every day is becoming one of those days for you, Kathleen. You better watch it."

"Wow, that hurts," Kathleen said. "Maybe I'll call you Bitch Monk." But she softened the remark with a chuckle.

"Hey, listen. I'm only trying to help you."

"I know. You tell it like it is, and sometimes that doesn't go over well in the office, you know." Kathleen sipped the alcoholic concoction.

"What do you know about Pocono Biological Laboratories, anyway?" Jane shifted the conversation. "The place must be sitting on shit that they pray no one will ever uncover."

"It'll never happen. Money buys silence." She paused. "It's famous, you know. That guy, the one who founded the Pocono Laboratories, housed smallpox vaccine right where we work."

Jane drank her ice tea—whispering under her breath how she "wished there was a vaccine against corruption and greed—but it might wipe out two-thirds of the population."

They laughed and sat in the yellow light of the old tavern, with the clink of spoons and the raucous laughter of many of their co-workers, most whom they would never know, since they were of a department that didn't require college degrees, and therefore, little recognition or prestige.

Kathleen ordered another cotton candy-colored drink and ate only half her sandwich. The alcohol loosened her tongue and she began to engage the locals in conversation. An older man who called himself Hutch meandered over to the table.

Hutch was tall and thin, fit for someone in their late sixties, by the looks of him. He had thick white hair that fell over his right eye. The circles under his eyes were puffy and they gave him the look of someone who was always sad.

"What do you know about Pocono Biological Laboratories?" Kathleen asked.

"More than you want to know. I've been here all my life." He glanced away.

"Inside the Swiftwater?" Kathleen giggled at her own joke.

"No." The man grew quiet. "I've known about things; we locals have always known about things." He sipped his drink. When he spoke there was a tinge of stale alcohol on his breath. "They're still pulling monkey and horse skeletons out of the pond over there. Whenever they build, when they dig they find some pretty gruesome stuff. Do you know Ron—he works maintenance over there—he could tell you some stories."

"Like what," Jane chimed in.

"Like the horse skeleton they found with three ears, and the frogs he's discovered with three eyes jumping around in that lake that is nothing more than a pond. I don't know who they're kidding."

"That's just folk tales. Give me a break," Jane said.

"I had a son. Born all deformed. Died before he was two. That's my proof." His words lay in the air like a mist no one could see through.

"If you really believe that, why didn't you do something about it?" Jane asked.

"I am a poor man. I come here every day. I sit. I stare out the window. I think about what my son would look like without his deformities, and how old he'd be, and what he might be doing. I sit here and I nurse my fantasies while I curse that company."

He left the table, rejoined his friends, even though he seemed all by himself.

"Everyone has to blame someone or something when life sucks," Kathleen said.

"Do you have children, Kathleen?"

"No. Never wanted them. I want to be successful, be my own woman, not give my life away to a man."

"Oh, instead, you'll give it away to a company that could care less about you."

"Connaught takes care of their own. Look at Chris Kirby. I mean, that woman has MS, and they haven't fired her yet."

Jane debated whether or not to share with Kathleen how she had been given the same diagnosis years earlier. She decided not to.

"Listen, Kathleen, I have to tell you something and you aren't going to like this either. Things are being said around the office. I think the boss lady has it out for you. Be careful."

"She doesn't like the competition."

"It's more than that. She wanted me to take you to a bar, offer to buy you a drink, and then accuse you of drinking on company time. If I were you, I would be very careful. They're watching you."

Kathleen stopped sucking on her straw. "Thanks for the heads up. But if you don't tell them, and no one can prove it, I don't have much to worry about, do I? It's their word against mine."

"Is it really worth it? Not sure I would play roulette, unless your job doesn't mean much to you."

"What a *fuckin'* bitch she is. What a bitch. I can't believe it." Kathleen stuck a piece of mint gum into her mouth.

Later that night, after dinner, Jane told John about the fish in the pond, the fish they ate, and the memo that came across her desk that morning.

"I wouldn't worry about it. Remember when we were kids—how we used to play with mercury, you know, roll it around on a piece of paper, hold in our hands. . . . The boys will be fine."

"I'm glad you're ok with it, cause I'm not."

"Listen, if you worry about every little thing, you're going to get sick."

"I already am, remember?"

"Babe, you've always been a justice seeker. You're the only one in your family that stood up to your dad. But not everyone is against you. You don't have to fight every battle."

"So, I'm just supposed to close my eyes and leave all this shit alone."

"Hey, you know what the priests taught us—there is poetic justice."

"Yea, and if you remember, cause I pass the courthouse every day, that there is a scale, weighing the good and the bad. When that scale tilts one way or another. . . . "

"Give it up, Babe. You'll drive yourself crazy."

"Maybe I'll go crazier if I don't do anything about it."

That night, lying in bed while John took a shower, she thought about the scales of justice. The goddess, whoever she was in ancient mythology, with a scale in one hand, a sword in the other. She imagined the sword a syringe and the blindfold pulled tight around the eyes. That was what it felt like, this company culture, a blindfold pulled so tight all one saw was imaginary light.

CHAPTER SIX

"A Company . . . No Better Than the People Behind Them"

—— ⚉ ——

"As they say, a company and its products are no better than the people behind them," the pharmacist from Juneau, Alaska, wrote. He had ordered one 10 ml vial of inactivated polio. "My request was handled first class by a woman named Jane. She was courteous, knowledgeable, friendly, and articulate." The adjectives flowed from the paper, to her hand, to beneath her skin.

> Living in Southwest Alaska, where everything comes in by water or air, can sometimes be a headache as far as trying to get something in a timely manner. I felt as if I was dealing with someone next door. . . . It was a fifty dollar order that received a million dollars worth of service.

Juneau, Alaska—a far cry from home, a far reach—and she, Jane Gagliardo, had made a difference thousands of miles away. In her cubical, she sat and leaned her head back, craning her neck toward the ceiling that seemed as if it was the sky itself.

A few weeks later, Jane overheard Alice talking to McCoy about the telemarketing company that Connaught had hired to the tune of hundreds of thousands of dollars to sell their products. When McCoy sauntered back into his office, Jane knocked on his open door. He nodded toward her to enter.

"Listen, I have an idea. Just hear me out."

"Shoot."

"I overheard you talking to Alice about the telemarketing firm the company's hired. Why don't we do this in-house? It would save us a bundle of money."

"Well, it's a good idea, but we have no one trained, no department to do it. We wouldn't even know how to begin."

"Let me get some training and I'll bring it back to the company. We can set up our own department. It will be better all the way around."

"You'd be willing to do that, on top of your work? I wouldn't want to lose you as customer account rep. We're already down one person."

"I could work the morning shift until early afternoon then go work for a telemarketing firm. Listen, the other pilot program worked. We got our sales reps into offices all around the country by establishing relationships with doctors and their office staff. It's all about relationships. We could expand on that same idea—and if it's done in-house there's just more credibility to it."

"And you'd be willing to go out and do this for Connaught?"

"Absolutely, I love my job, you know that, and if it wasn't for you, I probably wouldn't have gotten it."

"Anyone else know about this?"

"No. I thought I should start with you. See what you have to say. Listen, I like challenges. I like learning new things. Why not give me a chance—what have you got to lose?"

McCoy was quiet for a few moments, staring out the window behind his desk. It seemed to Jane that all the management's offices faced away from the smoke stacks.

"We'll have to pass this by the CEO first. If he agrees, I'll work with Alice on scheduling you for shorter days, without loss of pay. Put a plan together, bring it to me, and we'll present it together to Dave Williams."

Days after Jane had plotted out her ideas on paper for the "new telemarketing department" and handing it over, McCoy called her into his office and asked her if she was ready to bring the proposal to Williams.

"Of course, whenever you are." Her mouth went dry, her tongue stuck to the roof of her mouth—her voice sounded to her as if it had undertones of tearing something sticky off a piece of paper.

"We've got an appointment in ten minutes." McCoy held a navy folder in his hand. "I've already pitched the idea, and you can fill in the details. He's got the proposal, so this is to seal the deal, hopefully."

Jane followed McCoy into a large conference room with an enormous table with about fifty chairs around it. The room was decorated with Connaught's colors—royal blue and white—on the chairs and walls; the table was a polished mahogany.

Williams was a slim man around five feet, ten inches tall. He had red hair and blue eyes and was balding—which in his case may have been a good thing since the red of his hair and the blue of his eyes clashed with each other. His shining head was a relief from the intensity of both. It was almost as if his looks mimicked the conference room with the blue walls and reddish table.

He had one of those perpetual smiles making him appear approachable. Why not? McCoy told her he was the youngest CEO in the company's history. His degree was in accounting; he had no Masters degree or Ph.D. According to McCoy, Williams lived next door to Dr. Metzger, a medical doctor on staff who had headed the company for a brief time. The doctor had grown fond of Williams, so he hired him for the accounting department, and so the story began on how he had risen in the ranks to CEO.

Jane popped up from the chair, reached out her hand and introduced herself—she wasn't going to wait for McCoy.

"I've heard a lot of good things about you, Jane. It's a pleasure to meet you." He sat in the chair next to her, not McCoy's. "I've had a chance to look at the proposal and it seems sound. I like the idea of no longer having to outsource our telemarketing. Jane, McCoy tells me this was your idea, and I am quite impressed with your dedication to the company, with your creativity. There is a bright future for you here at Connaught."

"I think it will save the company millions of dollars. Besides, people who work here are loyal. Telemarketers couldn't care less about their product. They only care about their commission. I think that gives us more credibility in the marketplace. People like to know they can call and talk to the same core group of people."

"You're quite persuasive. What do you think, McCoy?"

"Well, she's willing to get the experience. I don't see what we could lose. I suggest we put Jane in charge of the department, give it a few months and review the results."

"Sounds like a plan. Jane, are you up for the challenge?"

"I am always up for a challenge."

"I can see that in the way you look me right in the eyes. I like that in an employee—nothing to hide."

"Yes, sir, thank you."

After asking a few questions about the plan, Williams asked: "Do you have any plans to go to college through the company reimbursement plan?"

"My main goal, Mr. Williams, is to see to it that my children go to college first, and when they each graduate, then I will consider going to college myself."

Williams smiled, stood up and shook their hands before leaving them in the conference room. McCoy walked back to the customer account rep department with Jane and told her this was the first time since he's been at Connaught that anyone brought a customer service rep to meet the president.

"Williams seems pretty psyched about it. Good work. You make me look good, too."

For the first time in her life, Jane felt as if she were floating on a deep sea with no chance of drowning.

Within three days, McCoy called Jane into his office and told her that Williams had given his final ok on the plan and that he had been impressed with her.

"I suggest that when you take a job telemarketing, you find out how to put the physical room together. I will find a territory to use for the pilot program. Is six months enough time for you to feel confident to bring your training back here?"

Jane secured a job with a firm that was selling timeshares for Fernwood Pocono Resort. She was hired to work from three in the afternoon until eight at night. The work was exhilarating, speaking with people she would talk with once in a lifetime, and she'd try to imagine the person behind the voice.

At the end of the day, she'd fall into bed thinking this was her project, her baby, her child to send into the world that she alone created and labored for. If she could make it all happen, she would be indispensable to the company.

At the end of six months the company gave Jane a room where she began to set-up the first Telemarketing Department Connaught ever had.

McCoy was appointed to oversee the department. He told Jane on that first day, as new desks piled in, that Williams told him that she should get whatever she needs.

"If it means pulling people from another department, then do it."

"It's all about people, McCoy. If there's one thing I've learned in life and in this corporation it's, if you treat them well out there, they will be loyal to our products. The company is only as good as the people behind them."

CHAPTER SEVEN

Corporate Heaven

———∿∿———

TO: ALL STAFF
DATE: MAY 18, 1990

I am pleased to announce that as of May 21, 1990, Jane Gagliardo will be assuming the position of Senior In-House Telemarketing Representative (SITMR).

Jane has worked very hard for this promotion, and has proven herself to not only to be upbeat, enthusiastic, and easy to work with, but also an excellent Telemarketing Sales Representative.

I hope you will all join me in congratulating her and wishing her luck in her new endeavor.

CONGRATULATIONS JANE!!!!!!!!!

The letter was signed by Diane Turner, one of Jane's supervisors in the Customer Service Department, and circulated to all the representatives. The next day, Jane donned a new suit and a new pair of shoes that she had bought to celebrate her promotion. She looked in the mirror. One of her eyes seemed to wander off center, but on second look, it corrected itself. It had been seven years since that doctor had issued her death sentence and the words that were unbearable to hear: Multiple Sclerosis. Mind over matter, she said to herself.

"I'm really proud of you," John said when she emerged from the bathroom. "You have really outdone yourself. With Joseph in college, this promotion couldn't come at a better time."

"Yeah, I'm pretty impressed with myself."

"Come over here," he said.

Jane stepped into her new office. All the phones had been installed, the desks placed just as she had ordered, with a thick product guide centered on each. She was making her mark, climbing the corporate ladder. She, a girl from the projects, from small town Ohio, head of her own department.

The more she gave, the more she wanted to give. Connaught is as close to corporate heaven as anyone can get, she said to herself.

Within the first two months the telemarketing division grew to five employees. Telemarketers could go where sales reps could never reach, into the most rural physician's office or pharmacy. She built the department with five of the brightest customer service reps she could find. All were women, all were undereducated, and almost all were no older than forty. One had to have energy for such work, a sharp mind, and a strong ego. As long as they believed they weren't as good as their educated counterparts, Jane thought, they would work their asses off. Being a woman meant you had to prove yourself. Being undereducated meant double time in proving themselves to the company. Their weakness was their strength.

Often, for morale, and to build a sense of community within the department, she'd gather up half the telemarketers and suggest they go outside near the pond and eat their lunches on the picnic table. One day, as they sat on the wooden bench, a gray ash began to fall around them, clouding the afternoon light.

"Oh, look, it's a Connaught eclipse," Jane said, laughing.

The air smelled rank, worse than the usual burnt egg odor, and it so overpowered them they decided to pack up and eat inside. She wanted to pinch her nose against it. Within a few minutes they gathered their lunches and headed back, but as they made their way toward the office, the ash fell on their hair, skin and clothes.

At the end of the shift, as they walked out to their cars, they noticed the paint had melted away wherever the ash had landed. A memo crossed her desk the next day, as it did all of the employees, explaining that the company had received a bad batch of eggs and they had to be burned. Any car that had been affected was to be repainted at the company's expense.

The stench lingered over the campus for days and clung to everyone's clothes. *One can get used to anything.*

August 2, 1990: Iraq invaded Kuwait and seized control of the country. Within five days, the United States deployed troops to protect Kuwait's oil rich neighbor, Saudi Arabia, and call the deployment Operation Desert Shield.

Jane received the list of vaccines required by the military. Connaught was responsible for supplying influenza vaccine for all personnel, meningococcus for all troops on land in Arabia, rabies for the Special Forces, Tetanusdiphtheria, and Yellow Fever.

According to the list, the troops were being inoculated against diseases she hadn't even heard of, and the ones she had heard being discussed on the news: anthrax, the plague, cholera. She wondered about Saudi Arabia—how it is that such ancient bacteria grows in the desert?

She sat at her desk dreaming about the men and women who wait for war, their bodies teeming with every disease pathogen known throughout the ages and its corresponding antibody. And here she was—a nobody doing something that would bring the warriors home safe and sound from the minutest of enemies.

At night, she'd return home to John and her three sons. During those long months between August and December, she imagined her sons going off to such a war, and something within her sickened. Taking the military orders had begun to eat up her day and she had to scramble to finish the rest of her day's work in whatever hours were left. She couldn't stay awake much past nine in the evening, after the dinner had been cooked, the dishes washed and dried and returned to the cupboards. She'd fall asleep night after night listening to the television downstairs bringing the sounds and images of war into their home.

With everyone concentrating on the war, the mood in the office changed, as did the mood of the country. She ate lunch at her desk most days.

On the way to work she'd listen to songs about being red, white and blue, about being proud to be an American . . . "At least I know I'm free. . . ."

It seemed to her that the songs themselves were attempts to close the gaping wound still on the backs of Vietnam Vets from decades earlier. It was an outpouring of raw Americanism. Johnny, her middle child, now sixteen, would sit in front of the television screen watching CNN, listening to the newscasters interview soldiers "somewhere in Saudi Arabia."

Driving to work on those autumn mornings, listening to the radio and gazing at the flames of trees, she found herself deeply grateful for Connaught—grateful for the work, grateful that she could help her boys go to college, thankful that what Connaught manufactured would save the men and women from unnecessary suffering as they waited, poised for combat even as they played cards and wrote letters home.

CHAPTER EIGHT

"Replaced" May, 1994

Dave Williams, the company president, had reviewed the telemarketing department and reported to all the executives that not only had the department saved Connaught thousands of dollars, but it made them a bundle as well. He called Jane into his office.

"Jane," he said, twirling his pen as if scribbling on the air. "I need to ask you if you intend to get your college degree. I want college grads in management. You have everything it takes to be an outstanding manager—you've already proven that."

"I would love to go to college, but I have three sons that I need to get through college first," Jane said.

"You know we have a college reimbursement program. It wouldn't cost you much money, if you wanted to."

"But it would cost me time. As it is my husband is already working two jobs." She heard her father: *You aren't smart enough to go to college. Women don't need a college education; they're supposed to be home taking care of the children.*

Williams' voice sounded as if he was submerged in water: *You've worked hard, and I want you to know that I know that, and the department has been a great success. It was an experiment, really, that has proven to be viable. It's company policy that all department heads are college educated, you understand that. I want you to remain in telemarketing, Jane. I know it will enjoy even greater success in the future.* She watched as his blue eyes darted around her, as if she was everywhere but where she stood.

Jane felt as if the air needed to be sanitized after their meeting—bleached, whitened, sterilized, wiping away the writing on the wall. *Corporations didn't want women who put their families first.*

Two weeks after their conversation, Peter Marco stepped into the Telemarketing Department. He loomed over her at six feet tall. He looked to be in his mid-thirties, had dark hair, and was built like college football player even now, a decade after graduation—stocky, only with a little gut, and carried himself as if he had just scored the winning touchdown.

After being introduced as the new manager of the Telemarketing Department, Peter asked Jane to go out to lunch with him. A Last Supper, of sorts, she thought. Maybe she was one of the those throwaway employees she had read about . . . the kind that once a company has sucked the blood out of you, they toss you aside, now used up.

Peter appeared to be more passive than aggressive, soft-spoken, a seemingly non-threatening presence. Jane wondered if he'd be stomped on by the higher-ups at Connaught, if he had the stamina required for the department and for the company. But he had a college degree, one from Lehigh University, no less, and that was enough to make him somehow more qualified to run the department that she had created, that she had worked two jobs to learn how to do. Now a stranger was called in to take over.

They went to *Big Daddy's* for lunch, a popular restaurant down the street from the campus. At first he talked about Lehigh University, how he had been a football hero. Jane spoke of her sons and their budding high school football careers.

"You have children?" Jane asked.

"Yes, I have three. My youngest one is only a few months old."

"Three is a holy number," she said. "Your name, Marco, you are Italian?"

"Yes."

"So we understand each other then, don't we, without knowing much about each other? We're fighters. It's in our genes."

"Are you trying to tell me something?"

"You know what, Peter, I had the idea for this department and I worked two jobs to learn how to do it, and then I brought all of that to the table, so to speak. Not only did I create it, I grew it. A college degree has nothing do to with real life experience. It's a sheet of paper—it's like a marriage certificate. The hard work comes after and I thought that would account for something."

"I understand."

"Do you?" She could hardly taste her food. "I will teach you everything I know and everything that I have learned. I am sure you will be good for the department."

"Listen, Jane, I am happy to have the job, don't get me wrong. From the managers that interviewed me, you are highly regarded."

"But not highly enough."

"Their decision wasn't personal, Jane."

"The hell it wasn't."

Six weeks later Jane decided to return to Customer Service Department that she had left years ago, one floor below the Telemarketing Department in Building 45.

She felt as if she fallen from grace. Only a few faces were familiar back in the department. Alice was gone. There were more cubicles then four years earlier. As she sat in her assigned cubical in the corner, she stared at the partition separating the reps in front of her. She felt she was in a cave and it was dark and all she wanted to do was rant.

Grace Cooper, an upbeat woman, had become the new supervisor. She delivered Jane paperwork to fill out, including marking when Jane would like to take vacation time. Jane filled out the calendar, choosing two weeks in July, which was considered prime vacation time, and returned the form, along with the other forms, to Grace's desk.

"I am thrilled to have you back, Jane," Grace said. "You've always been an outstanding worker and you will set a good example for the other CARs."

Grace's height was enough to overpower any woman in the office. Big boned, long black hair, bare face—she was off-putting. She walked with long strides and heavy feet. It would be impossible for her to sneak up on anybody.

"I'm happy to have you back. Besides, we could use some of your humor. Sometimes this place gets a little dry, and that is an understatement."

Grace returned signed forms to her after lunch, including approved vacation time. The calls came in and Jane found herself slipping back into her "old" skin, one she thought she had shed forever, having morphed into a different creature, the kind with wings. She knew what to say, what tone to use, what questions to ask. She knew more about the products the company sold and the products in development than any other Customer Account Service Rep, or CARs, as they had come to be referred to.

Later that day, Jane received an e-mail from Grace reneging on the vacation approval. Another CAR wanted the same prime time, and since Jane had had a break in her service when she left to open the Telemarketing department, she had lost her seniority.

"Grace," Jane said, stepping into Grace's office, "it isn't right, and you know it."

"I'm sorry, Jane, it's company policy."

"Why should I be penalized for doing something that helped the company grow and expand? It isn't right."

"Jane, there is nothing I can do about it. I understand how you feel, but policy is policy." Grace turned her eyes away, as if to gesture the conversation was over.

"You know what, Grace, sometimes you just have to right a wrong. You know what it is to work hard, and you know what it is to give your life to this company. You went back to college and got your degree in business—would you be willing to give up the ground you had gained? I don't think so."

"Jane, we aren't talking about me. We're talking about you."

"You're my supervisor. You've always been fair. You've always been good to me. Can't you fight for me, for all of us on this? What they do to me, they'll do to you, to anybody, and you know it. If a policy is wrong, it needs to be changed."

"Jane, you are too idealistic. This is the real world. If they give you seniority in this department after you haven't been here for the last four years, it causes all kinds of morale issues for the other workers. So, your morale suffers—it's a matter of numbers. You, versus the dozens of others affected. I'm not saying it's right. I'm saying it's the way it is."

"I have never resigned myself to injustice, Grace, and I'm not about to now." Jane left Grace's office. She felt as if her balance was off and she shuffled her feet a bit to regain a sense of equilibrium. Tomorrow, she decided, she would tackle retrieving her seniority. Today she was dead tired already, and it was only two o'clock.

The next day, Jane went to Human Resources and requested and received a record of her employment history with Connaught. From there she went to her old boss at Telemarketing, Jerry LaBlanc, and asked if he would write a letter in support of her seniority. Then she asked Peter, her replacement, for a letter as well. Days later, letters in hand, Jane went about as high up as she could go, and left their letters with the president's secretary.

A few weeks later the matter had been settled. Grace called Jane into her office and shut the door behind her. It was the end of the shift.

"Jane, you won—"

"It's nice to know that someone listened, someone paid attention."

"Be careful not to use up all your favors, Jane. Just a word of advice."

"I didn't realize it was a favor."

CHAPTER NINE

The Fighting Gagliardos

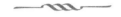

MS . . . the initials were deceiving; they told a lie, as if to indicate female empowerment. But since the S was also a capital letter, it meant something else, demanded a different kind of attention, relationship, as if to say a person was married to the disease. Why the abbreviation? Too many syllables, like too many complications, or was it that as the disease progressed the words would be impossible to say?

Short term memory was slipping further away into the dark spaces in her brain. No matter how hard she tried, it seemed to take longer and longer to fish out, to remember, to recall all the details of her life, which is why routine became more crucial than ever.

Such were her thoughts as she struggled every morning to get out of bed, attempting to tame the wildness of this neurological disorder. Her mental attempt to control the disease worked on some level. But she would ask herself sometimes: What does it mean when she tells herself her MS is under control? Whose control?

Every morning when John wasn't on the road, Jane would reach out to touch him. She would gauge the disease's progression by how much, or how little, she could feel with her hands. Long term memory always rushed in. Even when she couldn't feel his skin against her palm she imagined she could, and she'd close her eyes around the pleasure of it. Next test—she would force her feet between John's legs. Could she feel anything other than the pressure of his weight? This entanglement, this connection, she thought was the only way for the sheath of her nerve endings to grow back. Besides, what hurt him hurt her. *Couldn't it work on the physical plane as well?*

She spoke little of her pain, especially to John, afraid he might push her to cut back on work, insisting no amount of financial security was worth it. He would take a third job if he had to. They never told the boys of her diagnosis that had been confirmed by another neurologist a few years back, and she wanted to keep it that way.

"If you have one another, you don't need anything else," John said to their sons Johnny, Anthony and Joseph. He said it often, along with, "Family's first. You protect the family at all costs."

But she and John were protecting their boys from the truth.

"Is that why Italy is shaped like a boot? Italians always want to kick everyone's ass," Jane would quip.

"Hey, the Roman Empire never dies," John answered.

But the Roman Empire did die. Everything dies.

As she did every morning, she gave Christ a kiss on her rosary beads before leaning over and kissing John's cheek—the sacred before the secular she would say to herself, then chuckle, but never loud enough to wake him. When he was home, he usually didn't fall into bed until early morning, running the highways when the traffic was lightest.

She'd sit on the edge of the bed and ask God to give her strength to get through the moment. She'd repeat a few maxims: What you focus on expands, for one. Another, whatever this day brings will be a blessing to me.

Her feet on the floor, she'd hobble down the hall to the bathroom and shower. The heat of the water would help her stand up straight. *Life is good.* And it was always better when she made it down the stairs to the kitchen, placed a pot of coffee on, let the dog out, fed the goldfish, put on her make-up and curled her hair. She hadn't been able to feel the dog's fur in a long time when she'd pet him, but then she'd divert her attention elsewhere.

Sitting at her dining room table, the aroma of coffee wafting upwards, she'd thank God for the sense of smell and prayed she'd never lose it. With the newspaper spread out before her, she often looked for a cardinal like the one that came to rest outside her window that day of her thirtieth birthday. She left food out for the birds ever since. Watching the birds in the cold, perched on leafless branches and bushes, she thought how hard and challenging it must be to be a bird—weather, enemies, wind, rain, snow; the need to build nest after nest—wearisome tasks. Yet, she envied the lightness of their bones, the ability to fly, their beauty. Where do birds go to die? They were already residents of heaven.

Over the course of the next few months, the women in the Customer Service Department had warmed toward Jane, even the ones who had gathered around their computer and swore at her when she had won back her seniority. Jane knew they were really swearing at the company, but none of them could admit that. *The self is such a fragile thing*. They often came to her for advice on how to handle certain account issues. She had won their respect.

Military orders had become a major part of her work day now, and they were complicated. Connaught had to bid on the military contracts for vaccines, and then the company would have to comply with the terms of the contract. If the troops were called to war, the company agreed to supply the vaccines immediately. It meant big money. But big money also always meant a huge commitment to make sure all orders were in compliance to the contract.

All orders had to be shipped out within 14 days. Most of these orders were no less than $100,000 each. After an order was shipped out, another form was returned, about four-to-ten pages long that Jane had to further validate. About 20 such military orders came in a week, and shipments were sent all over the world to military bases. This was Jane's responsibility alone, along with territory calls, collections and billings, and customer service.

Her fatigued showed. Everyone noticed it. Sometimes the muscle spasms in her back were so severe she had to lay flat on the floor to ease the pain. But her evaluations came back superior that year. Such evaluations were like blood transfusions—they gave her more life and energy to continue to prove herself at all and any costs.

She and Peter Marco had lunch together once a week for several months after she had left telemarketing. Jane would bring in some sandwiches or leftovers. They would talk about telemarketing, its progresses and setbacks. Peter had established a new reporting system, and he had purchased new phone equipment. The department was flourishing.

Peter would ask Jane's advice, even though she sometimes suspected he really didn't need it. He spoke of his children, how his baby was crawling, how his baby started to walk.

Not long after his baby started to walk, Grace called Jane into her office.

"Jane, I wanted to tell you that Peter's wife passed away yesterday. She died of cancer."

"He never said anything to me about his wife being sick."

"I guess he didn't want people to know."

"But we could have helped, if we had known."

"She died in his arms."

"Oh my God, his youngest isn't even a year old. I can't imagine how devastated he must be." For a flash, Jane thought that cancer was like an abusive husband that lived inside a woman's body, beating it to death.

Why couldn't Peter's wife have fought longer and harder? She had children to bring up. She had a life to live, a husband to love and care for, pasta dinners to cook. How could she have died in the beginnings of their lives? Where is the justice in that? *You fight for your family no matter what.*

Peter returned to work a week later. Jane went to his office.

"Peter, I can't tell you how sorry I am."

He looked up at her. He was empty, like a shell she'd find on the beach, a shell that you pick up and position over your ear, but the sound of the ocean was no longer inside.

"Thank you," he said, and then changed the subject. After that, they never had lunch together again.

The fragile self . . . the walls we build come tumbling down . . . the stones others collect from its ruin. . . .

There was work. There was tragedy. There were military conflicts and contracts. There were miles of driving for John like all the other truck drivers, without ever really reaching one's destination. Destinies always changed.

One day in late 1994, Grace Cooper announced that a new building would be constructed on the campus and renovations started on Building 45. The department would be relocated to Trailer 8. She ordered them to box up their desks and report to the trailer on the following Monday.

Besides work, there was high school football, PTA, two sons in college, and the last son's senior year and final game of the season.

It was the annual Thanksgiving Football Pep Rally at East Stroudsburg High. Alumni, parents, friends, the band, and all the players and fans gathered around a huge bonfire.

Anthony, now a senior, was the team captain. He had his father's large frame, and his grandfather's dark eyes and olive skin.

Johnny arrived late, after practicing with his college football team— that year the team had made the play-offs and the coach ran them hard.

The two brothers leaned against one of the fire trucks. For Johnny, it seemed like the first time they had ever really talked without challenging each other to a contest of one kind or another, even if they were only conversing about the upcoming game.

"Big game tomorrow, hope you beat their ass," Johnny said. "You must be pretty psyched, being team captain."

"I'm definitely psyched."

"I'll be there for you tomorrow, cheering you on."

Just then, someone came around the back end of the fire truck and yelled: "Hey, there's a fight going on."

They both assumed it was a team member, and they turned to see what was happening. Johnny never saw Anthony move so fast. Johnny followed, knowing something had to be wrong to light such a fire under him. Thirty yards ahead they saw their father with his fists flying at some kid.

"Shit, it's Dad!" Johnny said to Anthony. "Someone's trying to hurt Dad!"

Never let anyone hurt your family. You have a responsibility to protect your family. Your family is the most important thing on this earth. You do what you have to do to secure their safety and well being.

In seconds, eight to ten guys started in on the assault, going after their father. The first kid Johnny came to, he hit square in the chest and launched him into some bushes. Another kid jumped on Johnny's back, and he reached back and over his head and threw him across the hood of a car, shattering the windshield. He turned around to find the next victim when someone grabbed him from behind and pinned his arms. Someone else was coming at him, landing a dead-ringer punch to his face.

Johnny turned his head, going with the punch; blood spurt out, he wasn't sure from where. He snapped his head back into the face of the kid who held him from behind and the guy's arms unraveled around him.

Someone else came after him and Johnny hit him once and the guy fell to the ground—three down, six to go. For a split second, Johnny scanned the parking lot for his dad, his six foot, three inch tall father with hands the size of baseball mitts. He was on his feet, his dentures loose in his mouth, pulling Anthony off a few of the guys.

A car screeched. The guys piled in the car that then moved toward Johnny. Johnny jumped in front of it and began pounding on the hood with both fists.

"You son-of-a-bitches, we aren't done yet!" he screamed.

The car careened around him and fled.

"What the hell happened?" Johnny asked his father.

"I saw this kid. He had his hand down at his side and it looked as if he had a weapon. I told him if he pulled out whatever he had in his hand, I'd kill him. I couldn't tell if it was a gun, but I saw this flash of metal under one of the parking lights. I knew, just by the way he was walking and looking at me, that he was looking for a fight. I still don't know what was in his hand, but he came after me."

"Did he have a gun?"

"I'm not sure. I think he threw something into the bushes before he charged me."

They scanned the ground, but it was dark and difficult and the bonfire intensified the darkness.

"Hey, I did pretty good. I think you guys did some damage, but I could've taken them myself."

Johnny looked up at his dad. "You're the one who told us never let anyone threaten the family. Family's first, forever. Isn't that what you've been telling us since we were born?

"Jesus, Mary and Joseph, what the hell's going on? I come around the corner and see all this commotion, and then I see the three of you in the middle of it," Jane said, attempting to run into the parking lot with legs half-asleep.

"Just call us the 'Fighting Gagliardos,' Mom."

Later that night, as John placed an ice pack on his face, he turned to Jane and said, "Our boys have become men."

"That's what I am afraid of."

"We always taught them that as long as we had each other, we didn't need much else. If one of us is down, the other picks you up and dusts you off and carries you for however long you need. Isn't that what we've always said?"

"Yea, but what would have happened if one of you couldn't be picked up?"

"We're the Gagliardos, the Fighting Gagliardos, remember? Together we're strong. Divided we're done for."

She looked at John's face, the right side of it swollen, and a bruise beginning to form beneath his cheek. Blood had dried on his cheek as well as a trace of salt that had dried white and left a path down his neck to his chest. The smell of melting ice filled the space between them.

"Your dentures were rattling in your mouth, do you know that? You aren't exactly a young man anymore."

"What was I going to do, let the punk kid go into the crowd and hurt someone? What's happening to this town? We have gangs now? Better that I got hurt than someone else."

She bent and kissed him, feeling the cold on her lips, tasting the invigorated salt. "You were quite a sight out there, let me tell you."

"Turned you on, didn't it?"

She was half his size, and he held her in the palm of his hand.

CHAPTER TEN

A Dry Hot Season

The Customer Accounts Department moved to a trailer while construction plans for expanding Building 45 were underway the summer of 1995. Trailers had been a fixture on campus for decades, housing various departments during numerous construction projects. Construction would begin within the year to add a $9 million addition to Building 45, the administration center, to be called Building 50.

Daily, Jane would walk during her lunch break to strengthen her legs. She had to get out of the constricted space, away from the heat. On her walk, she'd pass the stone house where the first office for Swiftwater Laboratories had been located a hundred years earlier. Inside: a high beamed ceiling, chestnut paneled walls and a stone fireplace; the walls were left as they had been decades earlier—adorned with guns, swords, pictures and memorabilia from the First World War. Swiftwater Labs thrived during wars. In 1898, the company supplied smallpox vaccine to the U.S. armed forces during the Spanish-American War.

She imagined the calves bleating as their abdomens were shaved, the skin cleaned and scarified, and the smallpox virus rubbed over the scarified area. Five-to-seven days later, the area would be covered with scabs. They were removed, ground with a small amount of diluents, and sealed into glass capillary tubes, or dried on ivory points, which were then used to scrape a person's skin to administer the vaccine. All kinds of bacteria grew on the calf since sterile conditions couldn't be maintained, and was found in the vaccines, causing infection in otherwise healthy people.[1] There had been a waterwheel in the basement of Building 4 that had once been used to grind smallpox pulp; Jane wondered if it remained.

A decade later, horses were bled for serum to produce human tetanus anti-toxin. The serum would be refined for its antibodies and then used to transfer immunity to humans.

Military orders had become sacrosanct for the company—World War II had become the proving ground for biological efficacy. During the Vietnam War, the laboratories increased production as they supplied tetanus and diphtheria vaccines to the soldiers.

She learned that four hundred prisoners in Chicago were infected with Malaria during World War II in order for companies to develop new drugs to combat the disease. All the inmates were told is that they were helping with the war effort—no explanation beyond that or the nature of the experiments. During the Nuremberg Trials, the Nazi doctors defended their own medical experiments based on these Chicago experiments.

Jane felt these wars in her bones as she strolled the campus, past the pond where duck eggs were once collected and cooked for the young men who came to work and live here. She was part of something greater than herself, that extended into the last century and was about to enter a new one. Yet, the lesser were sacrificed for the greater. Her gait faltered. She caught herself from stumbling over the smallest crack in the walkway.

Every time Jane walked the campus, she tried to imagine how the company looked back then with only a few buildings, no large buildings like there were now, no guardhouse for security. But the Swiftwater Creek still ran right through the middle of the grounds.

The smoke appeared thinner in the summer months, disappearing into the sky. Sometimes, she pictured them as the stacks from the ovens

---

[1]Jeff Widmer, *The Spirit of Swiftwater: 100 Years at the Pocono Labs* (Scranton: University of Scranton Press, 1998), p. 15.

from the concentration camps, and the thin ash that fell upon them the dust of bodies.

The trailer was a far cry from the dark coolness of that first office in the single story stone house. It was perpetual August, even in June. The air so stifling and dry Jane felt her lungs crackle with every exhale. She was sure the heat was on, rather than the air conditioner.

During the first week of June, Jane had sent off an e-mail to Grace:

I would like to make a request to have the heat turned down inside the trailer. The heat makes it difficult to concentrate, and I am sure it isn't just affecting me. Also, any news on getting help with the military orders—I am just too overloaded with them. We might be a department with the motto "One Call Gets All," but no one should have to do the all. I have MS and MS is one of those diseases that flares up and down. The heat causes it to flare up, as does stress.

Jane

She had difficulty too with seeing straight. Numbers were wavy, sometimes moving across an order form before settling into a column. Her neurologist, Dr. Peter Barbour, told her this too was due to her MS. Pain screamed between her spine and nerves inside her, but she remained silent.

E-mail from Grace:

Jane, could you please get a note from your neurologist that says you are under his care for MS? I hope this will be fixed shortly. However, I would appreciate you providing me with a written diagnosis of MS from your physician. Once provided, we can assure that your work environment meets your needs. You are aware that Chris Kirby in Human Resources also suffers from MS? Perhaps you could talk with her sometime about how she manages her disease in the workplace.

Within a week, Jane brought a note from Dr. Barbour. He had written on a prescription pad: *Jane Gagliardo is under my care for Multiple Sclerosis.* She passed the note onto Grace as she had requested.

Weeks later, Grace told Jane that the air conditioner was broken, but it would be fixed soon. The heat stayed on through the month of June. For days she felt as if she were being burned alive . . . disintegrating into ashes, scattering into nowhere when someone opened the trailer door.

It had been the second request she had made since returning to the department from the telemarketing division. Last fall, it was suggested that her desk be raised to take the pressure off her wrists, as her hands were numb. A supervisor from another department thought it would help relieve carpel tunnel. She didn't know that Jane had had MS, even though Jane's immediate supervisors knew.

It helped, but it didn't heal.

Each CAR now had their own *special project* to do, along with their other duties. Military orders were Jane's special project that was to consume only five percent of her work day. She was also expected to take 80–90 inbound calls during her shift. Meeting both demands was becoming impossible.

She had complained to Wayne Neveling, in upper management, who had conducted her annual review:

"I need help," she had said. "I can't do the military orders by myself. It's too time consuming. As it is I am coming in morning and night to complete them."

"How many hours a week are you working overtime?"

"About ten, sometimes less, sometimes more."

Neveling noted in her review:

Jane will log how many military orders she takes per week and how many outbound calls she makes regarding them. This statistical analysis will be done to determine if the military workload is affecting her normal workload and performance.

Sometimes the muscle spasms in her back were so severe, she'd stare up at the flimsy ceiling and wondered if it would melt and drip molten steel onto her.

CHAPTER ELEVEN

Crash, December 1995

—〰—

Saving lives was heady business—even if they were saved only from crippling or lethal diseases. No vaccines made soldiers invisible from enemy combatants or made them immune to bullets. Neither was there any injection to protect families from far more insidious diseases, rooted in unspeakable evil. Nor from crashes—the kind that changes a life forever.

The scorched air was especially pungent with the smell of burning eggs with the flu season upon them. The CARs worked at an accelerated pace copying orders, answering telephones, and managing accounts, all crammed together in Trailer 8. When the wind blew, they could feel the trailer shake and shiver.

Jane felt as if her body, literally, were emptying, one ounce at a time.

On December 20ᵗʰ at 21:38 American Airlines Flight 965 en route from Miami, Florida to Cali, Columbia, South America crashed near Buga, Valle del Cauca, in Columbia, South America. One-hundred-sixty-four people were on board that flight, and it was not yet known if there were any survivors. Rescue teams were being launched at the base of the Andres Mountains, searching for survivors.

Jane imagined the cold thin air from the aerial views of the wreckage among the jagged crests. Clouds moved over the peaks of the mountains like spirits ascending to heaven.

Why did such things happen right before the holidays and ruin them forever for those who lost loved ones? The newscasters' cameras scanned the airport—a chaotic mix of reporters and families seeking information about passengers. American Airlines employees had been dispatched to help the grieving families come to terms with the news that there were likely no survivors. *What would it feel like to be home getting ready for Christmas, waiting for children to return home, and then find out they were never coming home again?*

She wondered what it would be like for the rescue workers searching through the wreckage, the smell of trees and snow mixed with lingering diesel fuel and death.

Her beeper went off early Christmas morning. Gift wrapping was strewn everywhere. Her sons were rolling up shredded wrappings and whipping paper cannonballs at each other, even though they were young adults. Cinnamon rolls, bagels and fresh fruit were half eaten on the dining room table. The table had yet to be set for the family dinner; a ham was cooking in the oven, along with lasagna.

She phoned the distribution person on call, Mike Schlegel.

"We need a rush order of 1000 vials of Hepatitis B to go out immediately for the rescue workers in South America. You're on call, which means that we're responsible to make sure they get shipped out. I'm leaving as we speak. I'll meet you at Connaught in about 45 minutes. With the two of us working together we should be able to package the vials and send them out within a couple of hours."

"I'm working on finding a carrier in the meantime," Mike said. "They are all closed for the holiday. I can't seem to find one that will pick up, and it doesn't help that it's snowing out. Flights are likely to be delayed out of Newark on top of everything else."

John insisted on driving Jane to Connaught. Jane said no—it was Christmas. He needed to be with their sons who were home from college. She left John and the boys in charge of preparing the dinner. Her mother and father and her brother would be there in the afternoon for the holiday meal. *Burnt offerings*, she thought, as she rattled off directions on what to do and threw her apron down on the kitchen counter. John tried to tie the apron around him, but it was too small so he just let it hang loose over this clothes. Before leaving, she turned to look at her three sons and her husband in the kitchen and thanked God for them, safe at home, together, huddled as if planning a football strategy.

Snow was falling. The air smelled like fresh cut cucumbers. She drove down the same roads she had driven down day after day, but this morning it was different. Everything felt sacred and desecrated at the same moment.

No smoke was rising from the stack when she pulled into Connaught. The parking lots were nearly vacant.

Mike was waiting for her at the distribution center. He was middle-aged, vertically challenged, with a thick head of reddish-brown hair, and he had a "hitch in his giddy-up" as John used to say.

"I still haven't heard back from any of the carriers. I've been calling the airport all morning trying to figure out what flight this shipment can go out on. I pray we don't have to take it to the airport ourselves." He had already started to pull the vaccine from the shelves. "I feel really awful for those families, awaiting word."

"Yeah, I know what you mean. But it feels good, too, don't you think, that we can help in some way?"

He nodded, dialed the phone, and called FedEx.

"Delayed?" he said. "But these people need it ASAP." He hung up in frustration. "They told me to call back in an hour."

Jane was on another line talking to American Airlines about the order and checking to see if they had any flights out of Newark to South America.

"If the flight goes on when it is scheduled, about two this afternoon, we are going to have to hustle to get the order done," she told Mike.

Hepatitis B would be given to the rescue workers to prevent the spread of the infectious disease from the wounded and the bleeding, from all the bodily fluids that would leak out of the body upon death.

Each small box of vaccines had a number that had to be recorded in the computer, and then each box had to be packaged in a larger Styrofoam box that would protect them from breaking during shipment and to keep them cool to protect their potency. Expiration dates had to be checked. The smaller boxes had to be opened and each vial counted and inspected for any breakage. The process took hours.

Moving the boxes jiggled the vials, sounding a faint cry.

At about 11:30 FedEx called back to confirm they would be at Connaught to pick up the shipment by 12:30 PM for the 2 PM American Airlines flight out of Newark. It would be close. Since it was a holiday, not many plows were out. The FedEx driver showed up a little late, complaining about the roads especially in the higher elevations of the Pocono Mountains. All three helped load the shipment, and sent the driver off with the paperwork.

"That had to be one of the most stressful things I have ever done in my life," she said to Mike.

"No kidding. I'm exhausted. Let's pray it gets to the airport on time; otherwise the shipment may prove useless."

Her legs felt heavy, like iron, by the time she walked back out to the car. The snow was still falling. Her mother and father would be there by the time she arrived home, she figured, as she drove away. Holiday dinners were difficult, managing all the emotions she had toward her parents as she envisioned herself passing the potatoes, and cutting the lasagna into squares. Her mother had turned the tables on her father one day years ago when she had threatened him with a steak knife. Her father had called Jane from the garage to tell her to come and rescue him. Jane waited a while before she went to their house to intervene.

Violence breeds violence. Injustice breeds injustice. Corruption breeds corruption.

When she arrived home, her parents' car was parked on the street. She waited a few minutes, seeing their silhouettes through the living room window. To her right was her tenant's part of the duplex. A lit Christmas tree blocked the view inside.

Opening the door, she was waved in by the smell of ham and potatoes. Everyone was sitting in the living room eating crackers and cheese. Her sons were telling their grandparents stories. The room had been cleaned up and vacuumed.

"You must be important to be called into work on Christmas day," her father said. His temples shimmered like a splinter of silver in the lamplight. The lines around his eyes had deepened over the years, but his tongue was as blood-red as ever.

She wasn't sure if he was being sarcastic, so she didn't respond. Somehow, no matter what he said, his words always felt like a double-edged sword.

"Your father will be bragging about you at the American Legion hall this week, I can assure you," her mother said as if to tell Jane how to translate her father's words. The scars on her mother's arms were hidden under her sleeves. The one on her face had faded and thinned, looking like a thread that had stuck to her cheek.

She wanted to say, it's all a little late, isn't it mom and dad, this bragging about me? *Maybe I could have been a surgical nurse I always wanted to be. Maybe there is as much abuse in what a parent doesn't say, as much in what they do say.* Or maybe it was another form of abuse to keep blaming them for her choices. She felt as if she were searching for herself among the wreckage of her parents.

Jane gave them each a hug, hung up her coat and headed for the kitchen to help with the final dinner preparations.

Late that night after her parents had left and the dishes were done, she fell into bed and she watched the continuing coverage of the rescue efforts. She felt as if she was there. She would be in some way, believing the medicine had already arrived. Later it was discovered that the four who survived the crash were all seated in the same row.

It was also reported in the days ahead that scavengers took engine thrust reversers, cockpit avionics, and other components from the crashed 757. They used helicopters to go to and from the crash site. Many of the stolen parts re-appeared on the black market in Miami.

"How does it feel that you were some part of that rescue?" John asked her the following day.

"It's kind of amazing. I mean I do this every day, but I actually handled the vaccines and helped pack them up and ship them out. My hands will touch their hands kind of, you know?"

"Yea, I do."

"I guess you must feel like this, huh? Bringing truck loads of goods to others. I forget, sometimes, how what you do is so important."

A small brown dog was found alive inside the carrier in the cargo hold and was later adopted by the Red Cross team in Cali, Columbia.

"Strange, isn't it?" Jane said. "Then a dog emerges, as if a sign of hope. I wonder if that would have happened any other day but on Christmas."

A letter, written January 4, 1996, sent to Connaught from the American Airlines Medical Department read:

I would like to bring your attention to the exemplary performance of one Ms. Jane Gagliardo on your staff. Over the holidays
. . . when it seemed nearly impossible to get large volumes of
Hepatitis B following the air disaster in Columbia, this lady's
expeditious efforts provided me, in very short order, the vaccine I needed.

Perhaps as important as accomplishing this task was the
manner in which this lady conducted her business. She is an excellent representative of your company, who conveys through
her friendly, pleasant manner the good intentions of your company to serve its customers.

Please extend my gratitude for your assistance during this
time of crisis for my company and to this outstanding employee.

The letter was signed by Thomas E. Murphy, area medical director of American Airlines out of Miami, Florida.

Dave Williams sent a copy of the letter to Jane along with the attached letter:

Dear Jane,

After the hustle and bustle of the holidays, coupled with the
difficulties we are having with the weather, I decided that the
attached letter would signal the official beginning of the New
Year. I never doubted that we have the most courteous and professional employees around, but it is an extra treat when our
customers recognize it enough to take the time to write.

It certainly sounds as if you went "beyond the call" and I
wanted to send you my personal thanks. Keep up the good work.

Best Regards, Dave Williams

Jane folded up the two letters and tucked them into her purse. She
would hold onto them for the rest of her life.

CHAPTER TWELVE

Requests Denied, January 1996

The Whitewater scandal occupied the national news. Yasser Arafat's re-election as the Palestinian Authority dominated the international scene. A blizzard had slammed the Eastern states and was being blamed for killing more than 150 people. Three feet of snow had fallen in eastern Pennsylvania. Then the Poconos were no longer molehills, they were mountains.

Corporate storms raged as well. Jane wondered what the death toll would be.

Each CAR received a daily summary of the number of their inbound calls. A handwritten note landed on Jane's desk, dated January 6, 1996, about the same time Jane had received the letter from Dave Williams concerning her professionalism during the American Airlines crash in South America. It was from Neveling:

> Jane, we need a consistent 80 calls/day and hopefully the full 95 calls/day. Why are you consistently below 80? Since you are coming in earlier you should be able to make 95! Let me know what's up. If it's military orders, then maybe we need to split the daily amounts. Please review and talk to me. Wayne.

It seemed as if only minutes after receiving this note, Grace sent an e-mail out to all the CARs.

We are looking for a new supervisor to replace Brenda. Brenda has taken a leave of absence due to some health concerns. I am looking for feedback about a possible candidate. If you have anything to share about Judy Stout, please let me know.

Jane had met Judy when their sons had played sports together in high school. Thirteen years ago, in 1983, Judy moved into the duplex.

"Connaught is hiring just about anyone off the streets these days," Judy had said when Jane had announced she had been hired in 1987.

She was a plump short-haired blond, not too tall, about five feet, five inches, with blue eyes. She had a walk that garnered attention.

Jane had seen Judy on occasion around the Connaught campus, since Judy was working as a paralegal. They had exchanged thin smiles, a few grunted hellos. No matter where they passed, it also seemed to Jane that Judy was climbing invisible corporate ladders everywhere she went. What qualified her to transition to the department was the topic of conversation and the stuff of rumors. But rumors tended to follow Judy wherever she went.

When they crossed paths, Jane's mind flashed back to her thirtieth birthday when the kitchen floor hadn't been installed, the day she had been diagnosed with MS, when Judy had been her tenant.

After Judy moved out, the carpet inside the then-vacant duplex had to be torn up and the basement repainted. Jane and her husband used Judy's security deposit for the damages.

About a month after Judy moved out, Jane received a letter from attorney Carl Greco threatening to take them to court if they didn't return the $400 security deposit. Jane and John submitted the receipts for the repairs to the house and they never heard from Greco again.

What could she write in an e-mail—the rumored history of this woman who Jane thought had it out for her ever since they never returned the security deposit?

Jane had seen Carl Greco's name since she began to work at Connaught. He was credited, along with Dave Williams, in setting a new standard in the industry a decade earlier after a documentary was aired on television called "DTP Roulette".[1] The documentary drew attention to a study that had been done in the U.K. linking the DPT vaccine to encephalopathy.[2] Encephalitis, Jane had learned, is any infectious disease of the human central nervous system characterized by inflammation of the brain.[3] The special created more than a stir—it created liability lawsuits that almost caused the demise of the industry.

Faced with billions of dollars in potential litigation costs, insurance companies refused to cover vaccine producers, exposing manufacturers to risk and the prospect of bankruptcy.

Dave Williams was quoted during this time as saying: "We could not get insurance coverage and we did not have the cash flow or the cash reserves to support a self-insurance plan. Since vaccines were our only business, we could not simply stop selling or producing."

Dave Williams testified before Congress on behalf of the entire biologicals industry. He then went on to create the Vaccine Policy committee of the Pharmaceutical Manufacturers Association, that had since been renamed the Pharmaceutical Research and Manufacturers of America. Williams became the point person for the negotiations, along with the Swiftwater Attorney Carl Greco, who wrote major portions of the bill.[4]

Two years later, on Nov. 14, 1986, Congress passed Public Law 99660. The National Childhood Vaccine Injury Compensation Act established a government standards defense for punitive damages in liability suits. To settle claims, Congress also created a no-fault fund, supported by an excise tax on pediatric vaccines.[5]

---

[1]Jeff Widmer, *The Spirit of Swiftwater: 100 Years at the Pocono Labs* (Scranton: University of Scranton Press, 1998), p. 80.
[2]Ibid, p. 80.
[3]Ibid, p. 80.
[4]Ibid, p. 82.
[5]Ibid, p. 82.

The industry stood its revered ground, stating that the news media overstated the rare reactions and did not talk about the level of disease that would exist without the vaccines.

Jane had seen the miniature reproduction of the law in a Lucite cube on Williams' desk. Connaught had a better-than-industry track record in liability settlements, yet it contributed the same percentage of sales to the fund as other manufacturers. But Williams had set the standard for the industry.[6]

Jane decided not to respond to Grace's e-mail. It was an old storm that had raged between Judy and Jane that had fizzled out, she was sure, with no permanent damage. Better to keep her mouth shut and her fingers still.

Two weeks later, Judy Stout became Jane's new supervisor.

[6]Jeff Widmer, *The Spirit of Swiftwater: 100 Years at the Pocono Labs* (Scranton: University of Scranton Press, 1998), p. 83.

CHAPTER THIRTEEN

Incubation

Influenza manufacturing continued in high gear. Connaught required hundreds of thousands of chickens to produce close to a half million eggs a day—fertile eggs of uniform size. Incubated for 11 days, the eggs netted over two hundred thousand embryos for production.

And trouble continued to incubate for Jane.

"Your work just isn't up to standard," Judy said to Jane within the first few weeks of being Jane's new supervisor. "You aren't taking enough inbound calls."

"The military orders are hindering my work. I can't do all the orders and take in a hundred other calls. I have asked Grace and Mr. Neveling to consider giving some of the load to the other reps, but nothing has been done."

"You should be able to do both."

"If I counted the military calls, I would be way ahead of the daily quotas."

"You can't do that. That's special orders, not your regular work. Besides, you were the one to request the military orders as your special project, weren't you, almost two years ago?"

"Yes, but then there were only a few orders coming in. The workload has tripled since then. And last year they changed the procedure so now I'm responsible for making sure the orders are paid for—it's very time consuming."

"Are you saying you can't do your job?"

"I'm saying I can't do it all. Pricing has to be checked with the correct department; I've got to contact the military base to verify. There are military bases all over the world and they aren't all working on Connaught time, if you know what I mean." If felt like a war zone right there at that moment, a military base with a new commando on the scene.

"You must work on improving your performance, Jane." Judy's eyes narrowed as if she was pressing a trigger.

"Is there a problem between us, Judy? I feel like you're always hovering over me."

"You've been in this department the longest, that's all. I have to learn as much as I can. Figured you were the best one to show me. Besides, I skimmed your file and I saw that you have always exceeded expectations in your annual reviews, except last year, from October 94 to October 95, when you were written up for the quality of your work—you do remember that, don't you?"

"It's, it's just difficult to concentrate on my work when you are hovering over me."

"I'm not hovering. It's my responsibility that you do your work, all of it. Perhaps we need to have another evaluation," Judy said "I also understand from Grace that you have Multiple Sclerosis. Is that correct?"

"Yes."

"Could you get me some information, you know, literature on the disease?"

"I'd be glad to. Are you worried it's contagious?"

Judy jerked her shoulders back, straightened her spine against the chair.

"Of course not."

Jane felt as if Judy wanted to punish her for having the disease, for being imperfect, for reminding Judy of the frailty of body. What if Judy shook uncontrollably—would she still love her body then? Such simple statements—*of course not*—seemed to say the opposite.

"I'll call the Multiple Sclerosis Society that I belong to and have a packet of information sent to you. They're in Lehigh Valley, so it shouldn't take long to receive it."

"I'd appreciate that."

Before Judy emerged from the bathroom at the rear of the trailer, Jane called the Lehigh Valley MS Chapter and gave Judy's name and the address at Connaught.

A few days later, Judy came into Jane's cubicle.
"Did you receive the information I had asked to be sent to you?"
"Yes."
"Have you opened it?"
"No, your disease, well, your disease makes me uncomfortable."
After Judy left, Angie, another CAR who had a cubical next to Jane's, said, "I can't believe she said that to you. Your disease makes her uncomfortable? Unbelievable. You know when you're out of the office, she finds reasons to rummage through your cubical."

Around the same time that Judy became Jane's supervisor, Connaught started the Biological Ordering Program, otherwise referred to as BOP. The program entitled customers to order large quantities of products to be ordered and shipped at specific times to help reduce the cost of the vaccines. A field representative would bring the CARs paperwork from doctors' offices, and the CARs would process the orders from that point on, calling customers and confirming shipment dates.

Jane made mistakes. She shipped out an order to a customer on the wrong date. Another time, she released an order without calling the customer or documenting that she called the customer, despite the urgent request from the field rep. Late February, Judy called Jane into her office.

"Jane, you are making mistakes with the BOP program. Is this because of your MS?"
"Excuse me?"
"Are you going to blame your MS for your mistakes?"
"I would never do that."
"Then why are you making mistakes?"
"It's just a lot to retain. I think I need to be retrained—we weren't given much training to begin with. I'm just under too much pressure with the workload. It's like having to think about five different procedures all in same moment."

"I will have you assessed; that way we can find out what you're doing wrong."

Rose Kindrew, a senior CAR considered a support person for the supervisors, was asked to observe Jane the next day. For the entire morning Rose sat next to Jane and recorded observations, jotted down notes and later reported to Grace that Jane did not stroke very well. A CAR was required to stroke, which meant whenever a call came in she was supposed to press certain buttons on the phone which gave a report to the supervisors or managers to let them know how many calls and what type of call the CAR was receiving. Rose also reported that Jane didn't use Caller ID during every phone call.

It didn't take long for a written caution to land on Jane's desk a few weeks later when Jane made another mistake on the BOP orders. Judy wrote that she herself would sit with Jane and monitor her every move, and she promised there would be BOP retraining available as soon as possible.

A memo was issued from Judy's office a few days after saying that the responsibility for the military orders would soon be shared.

At home, Jane would fall into bed early, too exhausted after dinner and clean up to do anything but sleep. Sometimes she felt as if she were on that parade float tap dancing away but when she lifted her eyes, there was no one there to see her. There were no crowds, no parents, not even her brother standing next to her.

Her head ached with the sound of Judy's voice in her ears, like the clacking of her little girl tap shoes: "Your tone of voice isn't right. You aren't stroking right. You hung up too soon on the customer."

She was falling from grace, powerless to catch herself. Such powerlessness evoked a childhood memory, when her father pushed her brother, Dominic, who had just turned thirteen, down the basement steps. She and her mother hurried into the bedroom and locked the door, only to have it kicked in by her father, yelling, "I am going to kill you and then I am going to kill your daughter."

Her mother grabbed the closest thing she could—a hanger from the closet. She started to beat him. He was on his stomach and there was blood all over his white tee shirt. The cops came and pulled her mother off him, but she kept whipping the mangled wire hanger at him and threatened to kill him in his sleep if he ever touched one of her children again. It was the last time he ever hit them. But he only traded weapons. His tongue sharpened into a dagger that stabbed and sliced them to bits; only no one could see the blood.

Judy's tongue seemed to drip with blood too.

On Saturdays, when she didn't have to go into the office to complete her work, and when John was home sleeping in his own bed rather than in the cab of his truck, she would lie there next to him and not move. She would remind herself of all that she was grateful for, even the sound of his snoring, and the warmth and hardness of his arm under her neck, his other arm caging her small body. Hold me together, she whispered to herself on such mornings.

As she lay there that morning after Judy had "worked" with her, critiquing her every move, Jane thought about her sons. Whatever price she had to pay for them to succeed was worth it.

Their son Anthony was still home. He would soon be going to Fairleigh Dickinson University in New Jersey, about an hour away. Jane thought about his name—named after Saint Anthony, who was prayed to for lost things. *I pray to find the strength I have lost, and the confidence that is being eroded at work. I pray for my health.*

The cross on the rosary was always cold to her lips first thing in the morning. Her lips brought the heat of a human being to the metal icon. If she lost her job then what of the promise she and John had made Johnny—that he would be able to finish college? He was in his last year at Widener University in Chester, Pennsylvania.

Her sons needed to know they were smart, they were capable, they could change the world, and their parents believed in them.

Johnny, named after his father, would be twenty-one by the end of the year. He was a strong-willed young man who stood by his decisions and accepted the consequences of whatever they were. He was majoring in criminal justice and had joined ROTC. *He was a soldier before he was even a man.*

Joseph, their first born, was twenty-four now, named after his paternal grandfather, born eight months after she and John had married. He was a soft-spoken man, gentle in word and touch. He had graduated from York College in Pennsylvania with a degree in criminal jus-tice. One had to fight for what was right. The desire for it ran in their veins. Maybe the family genes had mutated over the last generation, fighting for those who suffered.

Sometimes she just had to take an assessment of her life, be an ob-server, and remember why she was working so hard to breathe.

CHAPTER FOURTEEN

"Just Listen to the Tapes"

The hard winds of April cut her throat like sharp slivers of glass as Jane ambled across the walkway. Judy had called a meeting. The door to her trailer-office was locked.

Judy opened the door. No one else was inside. The air indoors, in comparison, smelled like electric heat.

"Jane, I want to help you reach your target performance. I want you to listen to these audiotapes on increasing memory. I also have two videotapes on self-esteem and peak performance."

So, listening to tapes would improve my memory and help cure my disease? Are there any tapes for supervisors on how to improve the self-esteem of the employees—perhaps by dropping dead.

"Are you listening?"

"My ears are just fine, Judy."

"I listened to the tapes; they helped me. Listen to them in the car while you're driving home or to work." She handed Jane a set of tapes that were still in their plastic wrapper.

"Thank you, really. I appreciate that you want to help me." *I'm sorry, Jesus, for just wishing she'd drop dead a moment ago. Forgive me.*

"Chris Kirby, you know, she has MS. She's the one who thought it might be helpful, seeing that we have added new procedures that might be difficult to remember, even for those who aren't well, you know, sick."

When she said sick, the *s* whistled between her teeth.

"Jane, there is another reason I called you into my office this morning. Your performance isn't improving. Your mistakes are creating a lot of problems for those in the outside sales force. Millertown Pediatrics has been after the company for months to get their account history to them, and it remains on your desk."

"I haven't been trained yet in that area, Judy. I have to depend on the credit and collections department to do the history for me."

"I don't care—it needs to be done. They are waiting for the history so that they can clear up back balances." Judy didn't engage in much eye contact. Her eyes shifted from her desk to the papers in hand, and she shuffled them about, as if reading a list of complaints.

Can I take back my repentance, Lord?

Jane visibly searched for the packet of information that the MS Society had sent her—it was nowhere in sight. *What was there to say? Judy said she didn't care—about what? Or did she mean to say—I don't care about you? You, you make me uncomfortable; you, with your out-of-control disease.*

"I have sent out a memo that the military orders will soon change hands—we're going to share the orders with two other CARs. You should be relieved. I will need you to write a Standard Operating Procedure on the military orders so that we can have something documented in regard to what the duties are."

"I'll do that as soon as I can. Will there be a retraining session for the BOP?" Jane asked, reminding Judy of her earlier promise.

"Yes, I'm getting to that. Sometime over the next few weeks, I'm hoping. I'm writing up a schedule for the newly implemented procedures to be reviewed." At that, Judy reached down and lifted up a sheet of paper and never lifted her eyes from it.

For a second, Jane thought the paper was like a white sea, and the black marks, like islands, like islands of exile. She would feel it in the air—this punishment, even before Judy spoke.

"You're on probation. The Company has to take the next step in the disciplinary process, which is formal probation. Do you understand that you'll be on four weeks probation starting today? If you make any errors during this time, your employment with Connaught may be terminated? I need you to sign here."

Probation? I've been here almost ten years and you're putting me on probation? She braced her knees, tightened her fist.

"You can't be serious, probation? Have I made that many mistakes that you have to put me on probation?"

"Just sign the paper, Jane."

"I can't believe this."

"It really shouldn't come as that much of a surprise. After all, there has been a whole litany of mistakes."

The only mistake made here is that they made you my supervisor.

"I love my job, Judy."

"But you can't seem to do it."

Jane signed and dated the documentation, April 16th, 1996. She was rowing toward the islands of exile, and there was nothing she could do about it.

That night, before driving out of the parking lot, she opened up the set of cassette tapes and placed the first one into the tape deck. *Please, God, help me to do better. Please help me not to lose my job.*

"First, before you begin, you will need paper and a pencil to write things down for all the lessons contained in this Improve Your Memory cassette tape set."

"That son-of-a-bitch. Do they have any tapes for someone suffering from asshole-ism? Had she even listened to the tapes herself as she said she had?" she muttered to herself.

Jane listened to the voice on the tape, unable to write anything down as she drove. Her hands were trembling as if she were writing stuff down on her bones.

The next morning she asked Judy, "Were the same tapes you gave me the same ones you listened to?"

"Well, I really didn't have the time to listen to them."

"Since the tapes require a fair amount of work, could I listen to them on company time, since it is supposed to help me do my job?"

"Your function," Judy answered, her voice pitched higher, and the straight lines above her upper lip more pronounced as she puckered her mouth as if she were about to spit, "in case you forgot, is to answer the phones and do the military orders. You listen to the tapes on your own time!"

The government had just awarded Connaught marketing authorization for Hepatitis A vaccine. Jane read up about the disease and the vaccine at home, so she'd be ready when calls came in.

Hepatitis A: 1.5 million cases a year . . . only humans carried it . . . infection of the liver . . . through fecal-oral route . . . usually through contact with an infected person or eating or drinking contaminated food.

She read an article in the newspaper about the Operation Desert Storm Vets suffering from what was being called the Gulf War Syndrome. Symptoms included chronic fatigue, loss of muscle control, headaches, dizziness, loss of balance, memory problems, muscle and joint pain. . . .

The report went on—during Operation Desert Storm, 41 percent of US combat soldiers and 57–75 percent of UK soldiers were vaccinated against anthrax—even though the vaccine never went through large scale clinical trials—and many of the soldiers were suffering effects that some thought were related to the vaccine.

Her head throbbed with a familiar fear—what if the very company she was working for, the very company that ran in her veins, and maybe even in her water, was making her sick? She sat at her kitchen table, the dishes washed and air drying, the smells of fried chicken still hanging in the air, and placed the pile of material in front of her. Anthony was in bed, and John wasn't home yet. She remembered old files that she had stored away in a box in the laundry room about how vaccines had been made by various companies. She dug them out to study them . . . the Imovax Rabies vaccine contained aborted fetal tissue. The polio vaccine contained the 2-phenoxyethenol continuous line of monkey kidney cells.[1]

The first effective polio vaccine was developed in 1952 by Jonas Salk, but eighteen years earlier a research assistant at New York Uni-

---

[1] www.FDA.gov/downloads/biologicsbloodvaccines/approvedproducts/ucm133479.pdf
.

versity attempted to produce a polio vaccine from ground-up monkey spinal cords.

Then the woman's voice—the voice of the young mother who had called her not long after she was first employed—screeched in her head like a caged monkey—*you killed my baby, you killed my baby*. DPT— pertussis portion, created in 1912 consisted of B. pertussis bacteria killed with heat, preserved with formaldehyde and injected into children. In the early 1940's, aluminum was added as a drug-enhancing agent and later the mercury preservative, thimerosal, was added when pertussis was combined with diphtheria and tetanus.

Jane went to the computer and started to research more information. It was reported in 1933 that two babies died within minutes of the vaccination; others were brain damaged. In 1948, a doctor warned that children suffered brain inflammation within 72 hours of receiving the vaccine. In a later research in 1981, it was reported that 1 in 875 DPT shots had the adverse effect of convulsion or shock within 48 hours of vaccination.

She was born in 1953—before they knew what they were discovering now. What about Alzheimer's disease? Maybe vaccine makers ruled the world from the inside out.

Or maybe paranoia was a symptom of MS. Maybe MS stood for "**M**aladjusted **S**yndrome" or "**M**istrust & **S**uspicion" . . . or maybe the M stood for Metals and S for System—**M**etals in her **S**ystem, she thought.

She then searched for more information on Multiple Sclerosis trying to find herself. Symptoms included becoming overwhelmed when confronted with something too complex, short term memory problems, inability to maintain focus on a task, and slower rate of processing information, slower than those without the disease.

But she wouldn't and couldn't blame her troubles at work on her MS. . . . MS would not win this battle. If only they would finally give the military orders away. If only she could do what she was hired to do, without Judy's intimidation.

Injustice had to be fought on its own turf, she decided. The injustice of her disease was the hardest one of all to fight.

Chris Kirby called, requesting a private meeting. It was in the early afternoon and the day was warm and sunny. Jane headed toward a conference room that had been set up in a different trailer. She had only been on probation for three days.

"Chris, you wanted to see me?"

They were alone.

Chris was in her wheelchair beneath a window that left her features in shadow until Jane's eyes adjusted to the change of light.

"Yes. I wanted a pri-private conversation with you—I wanted to ask you a question."

"Are you tape recording this meeting?"

"No, Jane." Chris bent her head and shook it as if in disbelief. "You don't need to be so paranoid. I wanted a private meeting with you for one reason. I want you to know if you are aware of how serious the errors are that you're making?"

"How can I not? Judy keeps reminding me. Every day she's been on top of me like a dog in heat, taunting me every minute, telling me what I'm doing wrong. It's impossible to function when someone's doing that to you. And she isn't doing it to the other CARs either. Come over and see what I'm saying's true. I can't think straight. I feel like she is setting me up to fall and giving me a push all at the same time."

"Do you think that your MS is interfering with your ability to do your job?" Chris' hands were on her wheels and she was rocking back and forth gently as if to comfort herself.

"I think it might be. When I'm under pressure and intense scrutiny, I can't seem to do my job. I'm constantly being watched and told every moment of everyday what I am doing wrong, be it something small or large. It's overwhelming."

"MS is a strange disease, Jane. One day I can't get out of the wheelchair; the next day I feel as if I don't need it at all."

"Maybe it's my MS, or maybe it's just the way anyone would react if they were under constant scrutiny."

"I understand it would be difficult to be put under a microscope like that. But do you think it is more difficult because of your MS?"

"I don't know. Yes, I guess." Jane looked down at the soiled carpet and then straight at Chris. "Does MS ever affect your work performance?"

"It affects your life, all of it, your relationships, how you think about yourself, everything." Chris had a look to her face and if she were looking at a mirror reflection.

Jane was sure she saw tears in Chris' eyes. She sniffled, wiped her nose with a tissue that had been balled up in her hand. She didn't talk for about a minute, as if reassembling a dam behind her eyes.

Then she said: "Your errors have been costly to the company. If you need something let me know."

A group of people barged into the room, interrupted the meeting. Chris bowed her head, turned and wheeled herself away from Jane.

CHAPTER FIFTEEN

"Just Sign Here"

Jane sat at her dining room table sipping a cup of coffee. The windows were opened. Warm mid-May evening breezes scented with lilacs blew over her face. She clutched the rosary in her left hand that trembled, pressed the beads into her palm until they dented her flesh. How much longer could she endure Judy's micromanaging her work?

It was late by the time John came home through the back door as he always did so as not to track in the house all the grime of the world on the soles of his shoes. She had fallen asleep waiting for him upstairs in the bedroom. She heard him in the kitchen, the refrigerator door opening, shutting, and the clunk of something being placed on the counter. Too exhausted to get up, she lay there expecting him to come upstairs soon.

Ten minutes passed. John came into the bedroom and shut the door behind him, undressed, and left his clothes in a heap on the floor.

She could smell the road on him—dust, sweat, fuel, cigarette smoke.

He sat on the edge of the bed.

"You awake?" he asked.

"Yeah." She rubbed her eyes and looked at him. "You've been working too hard. I know being on the road is a hard way to make a living."

His skin seemed grayish—maybe that was the way he always came home. Maybe she wasn't awake enough to see straight, or maybe it was because he hadn't showered yet. Hot water would draw the pink up into his sallow skin. Maybe it was the sting of the light in her eyes.

"I love my job, John; you know I do. I love getting up every morning and going to work, or at least I did—"

"I know, Babe. I know. But work's been taking its toll on you, never mind how humiliating it is for the way that Judy treats you. Don't let her steal your love for the job."

"I'm trying not to. I'm really trying hard not to let her."

"I know," he slipped off his socks and added them to the heap. "I'm beat. I've got 500 miles under my belt and another 500 to do tomorrow." He turned off the light.

"You aren't even going to shower?"

"I'm too tired."

He curled his body around hers and laced his right arm around her waist. Oil had embedded and blackened the edge of his fingernails, outlining their squares and having seeped into the hundreds of little gashes around them. Tar and nicotine, and every other inhaled poison on his breath, blew over her. It wasn't like him to not shower.

She grasped his left hand with hers and held it close to her, squeezed it as she had the rosary beads, to imprint his hand on her palm. His heart thumped against her back and she counted the beats until she fell asleep.

Things were looking up. A week later, on May 21, Jane e-mailed a message to Judy and marked it "URGENT: What is the status on the military collections?"

A week earlier two CARs were assigned part of the military orders, but she was still responsible for the collections, and the other reps called her constantly with questions on how to execute the orders, despite the fact that Jane had written the procedures up for them.

Judy didn't respond to her e-mail right away, but Jane figured she would in the days to come.

Eight days later, on May 29, 1996, Jane arrived to work at the usual time, around eight in the morning. Rhonda, one of the nurses on staff who worked in the department answering any medical questions about vaccines, was the only person in the trailer that morning.

Rhonda was tall and petite with long dark hair and had eyes the color of slate. She had a melodic voice. When she spoke, it sounded as if she was singing beneath her breath.

On more than one occasion Jane thought about having a private conversation with Rhonda about concerns she had about vaccines hurting more than curing, but she held back, afraid of possible repercussions, afraid that maybe the office had ears, even though she trusted Rhonda more than almost anyone there. It was as if Judy's suspicion and criticisms were contagious, infecting them all.

"Where is everyone?" Rhonda asked.

"I don't know. Maybe there was some kind of emergency that we don't know about. I'm sure if there is, we'll be hearing soon—just what we need, a little more drama on the job."

They both chuckled when a phone rang on one of the CAR's desk. Rhonda answered it.

"Where am I supposed to be?" she asked.

Jane could hear the voice on the other end: "You're supposed to be in the other trailer for a meeting with the rest of the CARs and nurses."

"Is Jane supposed to be there too?"

Rhonda turned to face Jane and soon after hung up.

Jane was sitting at her desk, trying to sign onto her computer. It wouldn't accept her password.

"That was Karen. She told me to come over to the trailer for a meeting, and she freaked out when I asked her if you were supposed to be there too. She told me to say nothing to you. I'm sorry, Jane, I have no idea what is going on."

Jane's phone rang immediately then. It was Judy.

"Nobody's here. Where is everyone? I can't sign on the computer either."

"Just come over to the office." Judy's voice was an octave lower than usual.

Jane hung the receiver up. She threw up in her mouth and swallowed the acid backlash. "Rhonda, I think I'm being fired."

"Jane, stand by the steps and I'll push you down them. Then you can get workman's compensation and they wouldn't be able to fire you."

"I can't believe it. She's had it out for me in since the beginning. Rhonda, I love my job. What am I going to do?"

"Stand by the steps, I'm telling you. Then they can't fire you."

"Rhonda, I can't do that." Jane slipped her arms around Rhonda and hugged her. "I know what I have to do. I have to face the music that Judy's been playing for me ever since she came into the department."

"A funeral march, if you ask me."

Jane felt a slight convulsing against her chest as she was hugging Rhonda.

When she dropped her arms, she saw that Rhonda was crying. Her tears seemed like the most valuable thing one person could give another at that moment. She wanted to collect them, save them as proof she was worthwhile, inject them into her arm as an immunity against what she was sure would was about to happen.

"I've got to go. Thank you, Rhonda, really, thank you. I am a survivor."

"It's wrong, Jane, just plain wrong. She's had it out for you. Everyone of us could see that."

"Then why didn't anyone ever speak up?"

"We're afraid too."

Jane's phone rang again. She didn't answer it.

She felt like a cripple, hobbling to the trailer. No one was in sight anywhere.

The sky was clear and blue. Even the smoke from the stacks seemed to float upwards in a column that dissipated as it climbed upward, leaving the air cleaner than usual.

Chris Kirby's wheelchair sat vacant outside Judy's trailer. Chris had to walk up the three steps to go inside.

Would I be in a wheelchair one day? What is about to happen is more crippling than my MS. She looked at her left hand and swore she saw both the rosary bead and John's hand imprinted there.

Judy was finally going to collect her four hundred dollar rental deposit.

Jane knocked on the locked door.

Judy answered, opening the door. "Come in and sit down."

Chris was sitting in the chair next to the only empty one.

"Did I make another error?"

"Yes, and this time it almost cost the company the account. You shipped an order on a day that the customer did not accept incoming orders."

"The office was open though, right?"

"That's not the point. The point is you were careless."

"But the product was accepted anyway, wasn't it? The vaccines didn't go bad, did they?"

"Yes, they were accepted, and no the vaccines didn't go bad, but the customer called the sales rep and complained. That rep called me as I had told him to do."

"Let me get this straight. You told the reps to call you whenever they were aware that I made a mistake?"

Judy didn't answer. Instead she flung the order in Jane's direction.

"Once again, Jane, you were careless. Once again you did not pay attention to the details. It's too late, Jane. You can't say anything in your defense."

"It wasn't my fault. The sales rep told me to send it ASAP—he had a toothache and was in a lot of pain. I only did what he told me to do."

"Blah-blah-blah."

"Are you firing me?"

"You are being terminated."

Drop dead, you bitch. You set me up. Who the fuck is going to pay this year's college tuition?

Judy's mouth was moving but the word—*ter-mi-nat-ed*—came out in a thousand syllables.

Maybe I should have let Rhonda push me down the stairs.

A packet was shoved toward her.

"Sign the papers and I'll give you this check for $10,000, a thousand dollars for every year you have been with the company. It's the company's way of thanking you for all your hard work." Judy opened the packet. "Here, just sign here."

"I'm not going to sign anything until my lawyer looks it over."

"Listen here." Judy's voice raised several octaves along with its volume. Her words came out all jammed together. "What-do-you-think? That the company is going to screw you over?"

Jane stared at Judy and then turned toward Chris. "You're kidding, right? Trust the company? You just fired me and now you want me to trust you and sign a document that I haven't even looked at?"

Chris spoke up for the first time. "Jane, just sign the papers. It will make everyone's life easier. If you sign the papers saying that you are re-signing, the company will send you to a service that will help you draw up a resume and help you find another job. If you sign, you'll also get vacation pay, but you won't be able to file for unemployment until your pay is completed, and that wouldn't be for six months. Do you understand? You'll have the chance to save some money and get professional advice for another job, but I doubt you will ever get a position as good as this one. Let's face it, you really aren't that qualified."

"After I show the papers to my lawyer, then we will have a conversation about whether signing will make life easier for everyone."

Judy stepped away from her desk and began to make copies of the papers.

Chris' entire body shivered as if she were suddenly cold. She couldn't seem to stop it.

"Chris, are you ok?" Jane asked. "Maybe you should drink some water or something." *You don't believe a word you are saying, do you? How could you turn on me, too? We fight a common enemy, and you turn on me?*

She shook her head. With each shiver it looked as if she were inching herself out of the chair and was about to fall on the floor.

"This conversation is over." Judy handed Jane a copy of the papers. "You need to collect your things."

"Is security going to escort me out?"

"No. I want to give you some dignity."

Dignity? You're shitting all over me again.

Judy moved toward the door and opened it after she seemed to pull out of nowhere an empty box, the kind the company shipped vaccines in—was that intentional—a reminder of her so called crime? She waited for Jane to walk through it, one last time.

"Dead men walking" were the only words circling in Jane's head as she entered the CAR trailer. Rhonda was gone.

"Where are the other CARs?"

"I didn't want to embarrass you by having your co-workers present."

"I'm not the one who should be embarrassed."

Judy dropped the box at Jane's feet. It looked like a small casket that Jane's entire body could fit in.

Jane placed inside it two photographs, literature about the vaccines that she prayed Judy wouldn't inquire about since it was sealed in a manila envelope, and her lunch that she had packed so she could work at her desk during lunch break.

"This isn't personal, Jane."

"The hell it isn't."

Judy said nothing as she escorted Jane to her car. She yanked off her parking tags that hung next to her handicap tag.

"You need to leave the compound now. Security has been notified."

A half mile down the road Jane pulled the car over. She leaned her head against the steering wheel. Why didn't MS cut off the nerve impulse of the things that hurt the most?

"Sweet Jesus, what am I going to do? How am I going to tell my family? How am I going to tell my parents that I was fired? How am I going to face my kids? I'm so ashamed."

And she wept.

CHAPTER SIXTEEN

Guilty Innocence

———∞———

The packet shifted around the front seat as she drove up Route 611, a bumpy road like most roads in Pennsylvania, too long neglected. She couldn't go home. She drove toward her parents' home in Pocono Lake, remembering the day her father signed the papers that ruined his life.

They had moved out of the projects in Warren and into a brand new house that her father had built along with friends and relatives, in Levittsburg, about a half-hour drive away from where she had spent the first eight years of her life. She missed the projects, the impromptu picnics with the black family who lived there too, fishing with one of her neighbors, Moses, in the Mahoney River, not far from the apartment building. There were always playmates and places she imagined she could run away to.

Her father used his GI bill to build the house in this rural and seemingly safe community. The family had lived in the basement of the house under construction for two years before the upstairs was finished.

It was May, 1963. Jane had just settled into her new room. For the first time in her life she heard birds singing. School had just let out and she and Dominic were watching television.

As usual, her mother was kneading dough in the kitchen when the doorbell rang.

"Can I help you?" her mother asked, opening the door to two men dressed in business suits, white shirts, thin ties.

Jane wondered if they were the *Fuller Brush Men*, but they didn't have any suitcase in hand, and they usually didn't come in twos.

"Is this the residence of Chester Dovidio?"

"Yes. Who's asking?" She wiped her flour covered hands on her apron.

"The FBI, madam," and they both, as if rehearsed, flashed their identification cards and badges at the same time. "Are you Elizabeth Dovidio, wife of Chester Dovidio?"

"Yes."

"Is Mr. Dovidio home?"

But her father hadn't hit her Mom in days . . . were the police finally going to haul his ass in? Didn't they know that her parents were in the honeymoon stage right now, and the beatings wouldn't start again for at least another month?

"No, he's working. Would you like to come in and wait for him? I have some coffee cake that is about to come out of the oven in a few minutes. I could brew you some coffee." She waved them inside.

It was as if they didn't hear her invitation. "We believe your husband has stolen a piece of property from the steel mill."

"What does it look like?"

"It's a large piece of equipment used to help bend very large pipes. May we look around?"

"Yes, of course. I'm sure my husband hasn't stolen anything. Dominic, Janie, show these gentlemen around. Take them out to the garage."

She and her brother led the agents to the back of the house, out the rear door and to the garage. Jane pulled the large door up and listened as it rattled into place. The garage still smelled like fresh spackle and sheetrock. Her father hadn't finished the walls yet. A long machine was there, sitting out in the open.

One of the FBI agents said to another agent: "I think we found what we were looking for."

One of them pulled out a small camera from his pocket and he snapped several photographs, moving around the machine, photographing it at different angles, like an industrial mug shot.

"Thank you," they said to Jane and her brother.

Their politeness baffled her. She wanted to ask them if they were fathers. Did they treat their wives the same way? Their children? They followed her back into the house the same way they had left, through the rear door. Her mother had set the table with the Corelle dishes with the green flowers around their edge, cups and saucers. Coffee steamed up. Lumps of sugar gleamed from an opened bowl. Thick cream still swirled in a small pitcher, and the coffee cake was cooling on the stove.

"Madam," one of them said, "I believe we have located the stolen property."

"Please sit down. Have some coffee and cake while you wait. He should be here shortly. I'm sure he can explain."

They sat across from each other. Their stiffness seemed to ease as each plunked sugar cubes and stirred cream into their coffee cups. Jane wondered if they even considered that maybe the coffee could be poisoned. Sure, the cake was safe; it had already been made, but the coffee? *You guys aren't as good as you think you are.* These men were going to take her father away, finally. *No wonder mom is feeding them.*

"When is he expected home?"

"His shift ends at three. He should be home shortly."

The agents wore similar hairdos—slicked back, short, tight around their ears, with the smell of Vitalis hair tonic coming from one of them. Difficult to tell which one.

"Do you know how long this machine has been in your garage?" He showed her a picture of it, the steel mill in the background.

"I don't know, really. I don't ask a lot of questions, you know."

It was as if they knew then—their eyes dropped and scanned her body looking for bruises—was it what she had said, or the way she said it? Maybe they were men cut from a different cloth—as she heard her mother once say.

They could hear the car even before it came into view. Small stones had lined the driveway, and the tires made a crunching sound like someone eating hard walnuts. The agents waited for her father to come into the house. Their soft faces seemed to harden into a stern, don't-mess-with-me look—she had seen the same expression on her father's face, as if a presence came over him, a darkness.

Her father came in through the kitchen door and started to ask whose car it was when he saw them.

"Mr. Dovidio, we are from the FBI."

"What'a you want?" he simply asked.

"Do you know where this machine is?" The man retrieved the photograph from the table.

"It's in my garage."

"How did it come to be in your garage?"

"A friend of mine, he works with me, brought it over. He told me that he had signed it out of the welding shop, and he wanted to know if he could keep it here until he needed to use it."

"And you agreed, without verifying his story?"

"He's a friend. Why would I need to verify his story?"

"It was stolen, sir. The machine was brought with federal money to be kept at the shop at the steel mill."

Another agent drew a pair of handcuffs from somewhere on his body. "You are under arrest. . . . "

"Where are you taking him? Where are you taking him? You can't take him away, he's my husband, he didn't do anything wrong."

"He has admitted to being in possession of stolen property and he is an accessory after the fact. He accepted stolen property."

"But he didn't know—"

Her words didn't stop them. Her words had never stopped anybody. They didn't turn back. They didn't look at her or at Jane and her brother standing next to her.

Mom, now's your chance to get rid of him. Let them take him!

Her mother sobbed into her apron as she stood stunned, watching them escort him to their black car, leaving a trace of flour on her face that Jane tried to brush away.

"What are we going to do?"

Let them take him, Mom. We'll be free then. Safe. You won't have to worry about him hitting you or us.

Her mother picked up the rotary phone and dialed her mother-in-law, the woman who hated her, who slapped her across the face once for something she hadn't approved of. But Chet stopped her, saying, "She's my wife, and I am the only one who will hit her."

"She can't help," her mother said as she hung up the phone. She dialed her sister, who arranged to have bail posted. Their new neigh-

bors across the way drove her mother to the jail, since she had no driver's license. Jane and her brothers stayed home.

That night, in her room, with the door locked, Jane heard both her mom and her dad crying at the kitchen table.

"I should have gotten a lawyer. Our lives are never going to be the same. I should have never signed the papers. I gave twenty years to that sweat box. It was sign or be prosecuted and face up to ten-to-twenty years in prison. I gave it all up—my pension, my livelihood—it's all gone. I should have never signed the papers."

CHAPTER SEVENTEEN

Confessions

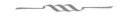

Jane pulled into the driveway of her parents' simple ranch home at the Pocono lake community they had moved to a few years back. Why had she come here—the most unsafe place on earth for her? *Just get it over with. Face the shame. You know he'll be a bastard about it. Maybe, just maybe this time, he would give her comfort, maybe the approval she was always looking for.* Chances are it would be like sticking her hand into the cage of a rabid dog. But maybe this time the dog would lick her hand instead of devour it.

It wasn't even lunch time. They would be suspicious before she could utter one word.

Confession: You were right. I am stupid. I will never amount to anything. Where is there to go when you want to run and hide in humiliation, whether you are guilty or not?

How dare Judy fire her! Fire—it was the perfect word for what it does to a person—it burns them up inside, and sets their life ablaze, destroying everything that seems sure and right, including any hard-earned confidence or belief in one's self.

Inside, her father was sitting at the kitchen table, the same table she had grown up with—a 1940's red linoleum and chrome table with six red-vinyl chairs. Just the sight of it, for a brief moment, conjured up memories of her mother's hands—raw hands from too harsh dishwasher soap, hands with fingers that were white and smooth and fluid when she cooked or baked. But that was ages ago. In the chrome seam around the edge of the table flour had fallen, hardened and yellowed.

The kitchen had been a sanctuary when she was young, as long as her father wasn't home. Fresh bread, cakes, pizza dough rising—pizzas her mother would sell at the church for a few extra dollars, the way her mother earned money for their dance costumes for the parade. Sometimes she'd see her mother punch that rising dough so hard Jane was sure it was a woman's punching bag. Right now, if there had been dough rising on the counter, she would have struck and hammered it herself until her fists were bruised from hitting the countertop so hard, turning the dough pink with her own blood.

Her father was reading the newspaper. The smell of black ink poisoned the air, stained his fingers; a smell that reminded her of all the days he came home from work after they moved to New Jersey from Ohio. He had joined a traveling construction company that was hired to build the World Trade Center. What a great monument to so small a man.

"What are you doing here?" he asked.

"Where's mom?"

"On the couch, where else would she be? Isn't that where she is everyday?" His tongue hacked the air into tiny un-breathable pieces. "Let me ask you again. Why are you here in the middle of the work day? What happened? Who died?"

"Me, dad, I died."

Her mother stirred from the couch and lugged herself to the table. Her gray hair flat against her skull. A white cotton-like film encircled her mouth. In the time it took her mother to stagger from the living room to the kitchen, Jane remembered the times as a child when she would come home from school to find her mother foaming at the mouth, lying on the couch, listless. Her mom had overdosed on too many Valium or a combination of Valium and Black Beauties.

That's how she remembered her mother—sleeping on the couch most of the time, always complaining that she didn't feel well. Other times when Jane would come home from school, she would clean the house, make dinner, and pack her father's lunch for the next day. The only time her mother would clean or move, for that matter, was when family would be coming for a visit from Ohio. Then she'd down some Black Beauties and stay up for two or three days straight, cleaning like crazy. Sometimes she would bribe Jane to stay home from school to help put the house in order. In return, Jane would be given permission to go to the Hullabaloo Dance Club on Friday night.

Black Beauties—her mother would force a few on Jane, but the few times Jane swallowed them she felt as if she had given her body over to some unseen stranger. There was nothing beautiful in these *beauties*, but there was blackness, a dull darkness, as if night had just fallen and she couldn't find her way home. Ever since, Jane had developed a phobia about ingesting pills prescribed by doctor or neighbor, even when it came to medication that promised to quell MS' ruin.

"What's wrong, Janie?" her mother said. Her pupils were constricted into small periods.

Why couldn't Mom have left Dad, rather than die a slow death in this marriage?

"I got fired." Jane started to cry.

"You didn't sign any papers, did you?" her father asked.

"No. I told them I wouldn't."

Jane saw tears run down her father's face—were they for her, or were they for him, she wondered.

"You better get a lawyer—they'll crush you, you know. They'll crush you because they can. You better get a damn good lawyer." The tears stopped. His face hardened.

"I-I'm going tomorrow."

"You should call HR and tell them what that Judy did to you long ago."

"I'm only going to do what the lawyer tells me to do."

Her father turned toward her silent mother. "What are we going to tell everyone at the Legion?"

You're fired, both of you, from being my parents.

Why did she even bother? All she wanted was a place to hear herself cry, to rehearse the words that she would have to say over and over again—"I got fired." If she said it enough times, maybe the stab in her stomach would dull.

On the way home, Jane held the packet in her lap. She pulled the pages out. It felt as if she were pulling a body from a drawer in the morgue.

Why were they so anxious for her to sign the papers—what would make life so much easier for them? She glanced at the words while driving. What were they afraid of—company secrets? Never say a word about unethical practices? Never confess that you knew where the bodies were hid—the mercury dumped down the drain, the FDA sleeping with the pharmaceutical company, and not theirs alone?

What about all the secret medical experiments conducted on segments of the unsuspecting population that went back a century—sometimes whispered about over lunch that went back to the same time as Pocono Biological Labs began manufacturing vaccines? By the time they were all revealed it was too far in the past, ungraspable, unchangeable, and somehow forgivable in the name of science.

She remembered someone telling her about an experiment . . . A hundred years ago, over two dozen children were used as human guinea pigs by a doctor who performed spinal taps on them, just to measure whether or not the procedure was harmful.

Then there was the Tuskegee Syphilis Experiment, conducted between 1932–1972, that had been exposed to the press recently. Impoverished African American sharecroppers with syphilis were denied treatment for the sake of being able to study the ravages of the disease. They weren't given penicillin as an effective cure nor told about treatment programs. The men died of the disease, wives contracted it, and children were born with it.

Thalidomide, blamed for thousands of birth deformities, was marketed decades earlier due to misleading results of animal studies.

Prisoners had been subjected to pharmaceutical experimental drugs and to dioxin, the highly toxic chemical component of Agent Orange used in Viet Nam. The men were later studied for development of cancer, which indicated that Agent Orange had been a suspected carcinogen all along.

For more than a decade after that, pharmaceutical companies conducted safety testing of drugs almost exclusively on prisoners for small cash payments.

Maybe she just knew too much, and they knew it too.

John was in the kitchen when Jane arrived home.

"Hey, Babe, you're home early. Did you have physical therapy or something?"

"No." She placed her purse down on one of the kitchen chairs.

"What happened?" He was standing near the sink, and turned the water off when she didn't answer him right away. "What's going on?"

"Judy fired me." Her head drooped. She couldn't bear to see his face. Her body slumped into a chair.

"She what?" John walked toward her and sat beside her. He reached out and took her hand and held it.

"She fired me. I'm so ashamed, John." She began to sob so hard she couldn't catch her breath.

"That fuckin' bitch."

"I can't believe she fired me. What are we going to do?"

'We'll figure it out after I kill her."

"I screwed up, John, but I didn't screw up that bad. If only she had given me what I asked for. She had it out for me, I swear it. I went to work this morning. Nobody was there in the trailer, except Rhonda—she wanted to push me down the stairs—I feel like I've been pushed down the stairs."

"She'll get hers, Babe." Rage blackened his already dark eyes.

"We have to be smart. Remember what happened to my dad, how he lost everything?"

"Yeah, but you aren't your dad."

"I made an appointment with a lawyer. Pat Reilly, the same lawyer we used after I had that fender bender a while ago. Do you remember? You never met him. Judy wanted me to sign papers, agree to take ten thousand dollars, and basically resign. So did Chris Kirby—remember I told you she also had MS?"

"You didn't, right—you didn't sign the papers?"

"Give me some credit." She stopped crying. "I'm going to file for unemployment. I'll get another job." Jane extracted the papers from her purse and slid them across the table toward John.

"I can't believe it. You've been there for ten years and this bitch comes into your department and six months later you're fired.

Anthony came in the front door. He was in his final days of high school and was scheduled to attend Fairleigh Dickinson University in the fall.

"What's wrong? Mom, what's wrong?"

"I lost my job."

"Does that mean I won't be able to go to college?"

"Anthony, we'll figure this out," John said.

"I'm going to try to get my job back, Anthony."

"How?"

"I'm going to figure out what my rights are. I've an appointment with a lawyer to discuss what my options are—and if Connaught did anything illegal."

"Mom, you do whatever you have to, even if it means I won't be able to go to Fairleigh. I could go to a less expensive school."

"We made you a promise, Anthony," John said. "And we'll keep our promise, no matter what it takes. You've got a scholarship for football there and it's a good school. We'll figure this out, even if it means I have to take on another job."

"Dad, you're already working two jobs. It's not worth killing yourself over."

"We'll find a way," John said, and then turned to Jane. "I'm going to take tomorrow off and go with you to the lawyer's office. Our kids are going to have the life we never had—including jobs where others can't shit on them." He stood up and threw the papers across the table.

CHAPTER EIGHTEEN

Patrick Reilly

———✺———

Patrick Reilly had always been a horrible loser—it didn't matter if it was losing a football game when he played for Washington and Lee University or arguing a court case. As an Assistant Lehigh County Solicitor, he had a few good cases that set him apart from other ambitious lawyers. So when he landed his dream job at the top law firm—*Gross, McGinley, LaBarre and Eaton*—at age twenty-eight, he figured losing was a thing of the past.

Allentown wasn't far from where he grew up in Old Zionsville, yet there was an invisible divide between the city and the small town. Center City's row houses leaned toward poverty and ruin. Don LaBarre said during the job interview that the firm had made a commitment to bring "revival" to the industrial-abandoned city. Outside the brownstone on Fifth Street where the firm had been located only months ago, prostitutes strolled in the afternoon beat. A lawyer from the firm next door would run outside to take pictures of the johns' license plate to scare them away—prostitutes and johns just weren't good for business.

Center City had already imploded, he thought as he drove through the rain. Even the courthouse, with its bone-like structure, was beginning to crumble. The deluge couldn't blur or wash the stains or smell of neglect away.

Passing the Lehigh County Courthouse, he traveled a few blocks west until he came to *Crown Tower*, the firm's new home, and pulled into the parking lot. *Crown Tower* was the city's newest crowning achievement and so named by the law partners. The building had been a silk mill before it housed a crockery store decades, and one major refurbishment, ago.

Inside, the entrance was a mixture of Art Deco and contemporary—granite floors, high ceilings designed with narrow panels of glass and stainless steel. He stepped into the elevator that opened directly into the law office. Above him, ribs of copper formed archways along the ceiling. On the walls, in rectangles of mirroring glass, he glimpsed himself in motion—tall, well-built, light brown hair, good looking.

Between teak pillars, yellowed posters told the story of McGinley's and Gross' family history in politics: "McGinley for District Attorney," "Gross for Mayor," a framed White House Christmas card signed by JFK, alongside photographs of McGinley shaking hands with President Kennedy, Gross' grandfather standing next to Babe Ruth, and a Muhlenberg College, 1894, football team shot where Gross' grandfather squatted in the front row.

Maybe it was the love of football that nailed him the job—the obsession with strategy, the killer instinct, the need to win. He thought of his high school coach, Fritz Halfacre, who had more influence over his young life than any other person other than his parents. Once, right before the first game of the season, Halfacre slammed his head against a locker, stressing the right syllable in the cry for victory, revving up the team. When he turned around, blood trailed down his face. He had sliced his forehead on the locker's air grille. That was the season of seasons—Pat set a high school record for the highest number of individual tackles in the history of Emmaus High School in the last game.

After, all Pat's father talked about was the tackles Pat had missed.

Four years of political science, graduating from Cumberland School of Law in Birmingham, Alabama and three years of practicing law were finally paying off. Gone were the days of bartending and being a law clerk in the good ole' boy South. Not bad for the son of a plumber—the son of a survivor. When his father worked at Bethlehem Steel as a steamfitter before Pat was born, an electrical shock from an uncovered wire caused him to fall three stories onto a corrugated tin roof that saved his life.

He nodded toward the receptionist and recalled the comment he had made only days ago, sitting across the mahogany table from *Gross, McGinley, LaBarre and Eaton:*

"For me, trial work is a sport."

The comment earned him a smirk from Gross, a nod from McGinley. They knew of him, they said, from the press; he had come recommended by a colleague. It was discontentment mixed with boredom that drove Pat from his county solicitor job to search out the litigation firm.

Don LaBarre greeted him in the hall outside Pat's new office, reaching out his hand for Pat to shake. In his early forties, LaBarre had salt-and-pepper hair and a receding hairline, stood about six feet tall, a few inches shorter than Pat, and wore glasses. As he led the way into Pat's office, he said, "Pat, it's your charisma, your ability to market yourself, and your legal abilities that impress us. We see potential in you to be a top litigator. You're quick on your feet, and you present yourself well. Your physical appearance, well, that's all part of it too." He had an infectious laugh that followed him like a high-pitched song as he turned on his heels and walked back to his own office.

This was the game of Pat's life; he knew it and LaBarre knew it. The only thing missing was a locker to slam his head against.

The new bluish-gray carpet emitted a trace of formaldehyde. Law books with gold embossed bindings glinted and winked at him as he walked to his desk and placed his briefcase down. Outside, the downpour was silenced by the thick curtain wall—rain his left knee forecasted yesterday as if the storm brewed first there, nagging him about past defeats.

Looking out of the one large window to his left, he saw farm fields shrinking with new housing developments. He had known such fields better than he knew the city streets. Growing up, he worked summers and after school, when he wasn't playing football, he harvested strawberries, picked and cut corn, and worked on a seed farm. Back then, houses weren't so large. It was the land people valued. Most of the houses, including his high school, had been built of brick, organic to the clay soil of the region.

His hands had never completely recovered from his early days laboring on the farm; he hoped they never would. He could still feel the sun on them, feel the weight of plucked berries and seeds dug from soft soil before they were dried. Each season the red clay dirt had a different smell—like a musk-like tang in fall, like wet shale in winter, like a swollen lake in spring. In summer, like deep water. Clay that seeped all the way into his arteries. . . . The land and its labor was in his blood.

Once he and his buddy Jeff had stolen a scarecrow and dressed it up in his sister's clothes, walked arm in arm along the side of the road. When a car drove by, they threw the scarecrow into the road. Drivers screeched on their brakes, certain that they had killed someone. Then he and Jeff ran into the fields to hide among the corn stalks and laughed until they ran out of air.

For a moment, Pat caught himself laughing out loud.

The trees were emblazoned beyond the cityscape. Old Zionsville was home once again—not far from the farm he worked where the corn stalks were pale and brittle. The apple orchards were almost all picked over by now. The sting of fermenting windfalls soaked the ground; he remembered how the soles of his sneakers carried that cider smell into the house he grew up in.

Those days seemed simple, innocent, carefree.

Would all innocence be lost as he defended both cops and robbers?

He remembered those days, as if writing his own biography. How would it end? Would he be a success story? Does practice make perfect in law? Would he one day be a rainmaker?

It was late afternoon when he called home and told Adrienne that he'd be working late. He had to prove himself, drive himself, without missing any tackles, he said to himself.

Her voice was more apathetic than angry: "Ok, I'll take Kristin to your mom's. I've got to work late this evening too. I'm closing a few deals."

"Ok, I'll see you later. Do you want me to pick up Kristin?" He imagined Adrienne talking to him from the stool in the kitchen of their small ranch. He heard two-year-old Kristin babbling away, probably straddling Adrienne's knee, her curly blond head resting against her mother's arm, her eyes a blue he lost himself in whenever she looked up at him.

Adrienne was still slender after birthing their first child. Her long blond hair would be flowing over her shoulders. She was taller than average—a knockout by anyone's standards. The color of her eyes reminded him of the Little Lehigh Creek when the sun lit the surface, more gray than blue.

"If you're home before nine, go ahead and pick her up; otherwise I will." She hesitated then asked, "Is this how it starts, Pat, you working late, setting an expectation right off the bat of spending your life at the office, defending others while you leave Kristin and me out to hang?"

"I'm just starting out here . . . be patient. I'm doing this for all of us."

"Sure you are."

"I'll see you later," he said and hung up the receiver.

They got married after his first year of law school, five years ago—a marriage that was not what he would call blissful, but it was comfortable. She had somehow always felt familiar, as if he had known her long before they met. Sometimes he wished marriage was more of a sport—with time outs. Sometimes it seemed as if there was only overtime—a tough game when there were no practices, breaks, and few wins.

They had met in college at a fraternity party; she was a freshman at junior college, he a football player with his own battle at "wounded knee." He had lost one scholarship to the University of Pennsylvania due to a torn cartilage. He was limping around, having injured it once again during a game for Washington and Lee, and found a vacant seat on the couch that spilled over with frat brothers since he was too shy to strike up a conversation, even with one beer down. One of the brothers introduced him to Adrienne.

"An old injury?" she asked

"Old and new," he answered.

"Can I get you a cold beer to put on it?"

"Yeah, that would be nice," he said. He watched her as she turned away and meandered through the crowd, a lithe creature with a subtle sway to her hips. John Denver sang out *Thank God I'm a Country Boy* from a stereo—it could have been his theme song. Cool Blue Ridge Mountain air breezed in and thinned the cigarette smoke. On the table next to him, a blue lava lamp cast its greenish light.

Adrienne returned with two bottles in her hand, and she wrapped one in a towel. She held it on his pained knee and handed him the other.

"Thanks."

"No problem. So what are you studying?" It was the first of many questions to follow—what did he want to do after graduation, where did he want to live. . . . He caught a whiff of her perfume, a sweet scent with an undercurrent of baby powder. She was studying to be a teacher, she said, although he never asked.

By the time Jim Morrison's *Light My Fire* vibrated through the room, she felt like land to him, and he like water following the path of least resistance. The lyrics somehow sounded like prophecy.

You know that it would be untrue . . . You know that I would be a liar . . . If I was to say to you . . . Girl, we couldn't get much higher . . . Come on baby, light my fire . . . Come on baby, light my fire . . .

"Not sure putting ice on you is such a good idea," she said. "I wouldn't want to put out any fire," she laughed.

Try to set the night on fire . . . The time to hesitate is through . . . No time to wallow in the mire . . . Try now we can only lose . . . And our love become a funeral pyre. . . .

The third beer doused his shyness. He found himself testing the waters, placing a hand on her knee. She didn't push his hand away. Drum beats and organ chords pulsed through the room and through his head as he leaned over and kissed her.

Weeks later, in his room, they made love. Her body was like the field next to the house he grew up in . . . with hollows and slopes . . . and fertile places.

He had come a long way, but he had so much further to go.

CHAPTER NINETEEN

Building the Case

John and Jane headed toward Allentown the next morning. They didn't say much to each other in the car, even though it felt as if they were having a conversation that encompassed their entire lives. They drove south along the Delaware River, a river that was at once rapids and currents, calm and flat waters. It struck Jane, as she followed its wends, how human-like the river was, full of undercurrents that claimed more than one soul every spring, flat waters that made you believe you could course all the way to the eternal sea. Yet beneath was an invisible world full of life and death. The surface was like the skin on a body, hiding the inner life.

"I think you'll like him," Jane said, staring out at the homes built on stilts on the banks of the Delaware.

"Who?"

"The lawyer, who the hell do ya think I'm talking about?"

They chuckled. At that moment she was aware of how it was that John understood her, how he knew how to decipher the tones in her voice, the inflections.

"I trust your judgment."

"I always thought I had good judgment, until now." She glanced away from him. Her face flushed. "I can't believe how much a job can make or break you. The job just meant everything to me, and now, because I have some limitations—it's like being given a diagnosis of chronic psychic pain."

"I know, Babe, I know. But the wound's fresh. It'll get better." John reached over and took her hand.

"Really, John? We don't even know if the lawyer will take it on, and even though I know there's been a great injustice, will he think we have a strong enough case?"

"If he doesn't, then we'll search until we find one that does. Some things you just have to leave to fate."

"Fate—was it fate that made me lose my job? This is the most humiliating thing that has ever happened to me."

At the law firm, they were directed to the waiting room.

"Feels like I'm going to the doctor's for an exam. It's awful to feel this vulnerable," Jane said, scanning the photographs on the walls to distract her. They were like the frames in a filmstrip, listing credentials before the film started to play—impressing the audience with great expectations before the first scene even began. "It's strange, isn't it, to ask someone who you don't even know to fight your battles for you?"

Ten minutes later, Patrick Reilly came to escort them to his office, and he introduced himself to John.

Patrick was in his early forties. His hair was just starting to turn a silverfish gray; he still had his "boyish" figure. As soon as they sat down in his office he asked to see the papers that Connaught had asked Jane to sign.

"They wanted me to sign them in front of them. Said they'd give me $10,000, a thousand for every year I had worked there. I didn't sign—I told you that. They said it would make everyone's life easier if I did."

"They should have said it would make *their* lives easier. That would have been the truth."

Patrick perused the letter, asked a few questions, and jotted down notes. He took deliberate notice of how John said little, sitting beside Jane, almost like a body guard.

After several minutes Patrick said, "Jane, I really don't know if we have a case. I will have to research it."

"They were wrong, Patrick. They didn't do what they said they would do."

"You and I can agree that they were wrong, or immoral, but that doesn't mean that what they did is unlawful. Pennsylvania is an employment-at-will state, so you can be fired, or quit, for any reason or no reason at all at any time. The question to be answered is whether or not we can prove that what they did violates the anti-discrimination provisions of the Americans with Disabilities Act." Patrick paused, shifted in his chair, and glanced at the photograph of his mother and father, remembering everything his family went through after his father had been injured on the job—he had fallen from a steel beam onto his back in the factory, the same factory where he had inhaled asbestos, day after day.

"Listen, Judy Stout, my supervisor for the last six months, told me that my MS makes her uncomfortable—that has to say something!"

"No lawyer will take on a case he isn't sure he can win. You're talking about taking on the most powerful industry in the world. Never mind one of the biggest employers in northeast Pennsylvania, if not the biggest. I'm certain that they have a team of highly paid and well qualified lawyers ready and willing to turn your life inside out regardless of whether or not Connaught violated the law."

"But they were wrong."

"If only it was that simple. The ADA is relatively new, and unfortunately I don't know much about it. Let me do some research and I will get back to you as soon as I can." Patrick walked them to the elevator and promised he would call as soon as he researched the case.

"Thank you, Pat, really, thank you for being willing to look into this," Jane said.

John shook Patrick's hand and nodded before stepping onto the elevator.

Inside the elevator Jane turned to John and asked, "What did you think of Patrick?"

"I'll let you know when we hear back from him. Sounded to me a little like this is just another case to him."

"I know." She paused. "Isn't he good-looking?"

"Yeah, he's so good looking, I'd do him."

It was the same dilemma that faced Patrick day after day—the law versus lives, humanity versus inhumanity, morality and justice were not always on the same side. He pressed the lower elevator button and watched the doors of the elevator close. There was something about Jane—a sincerity, a sense of conviction, an assertiveness, yet she didn't seem overly aggressive. She was the kind of client every lawyer loved to represent. And John, who may have dwarfed her by the sheer size of him, didn't diminish her in any way. It was clear the guy ruled the air in their home, but Jane was a powerhouse in her own right—he could see that when they were together. Patrick had something to learn from the both of them, and it had nothing to do with the case.

How do two people, who came together so young, manage to stay together? His first marriage was over. He had remarried to a recent divorcee, but he envied something about Jane and John, something he couldn't yet name, but he not only wanted to name it, he wanted to own it for himself.

A few weeks after Jane visited Patrick, on a warm June day, three hundred employees at Connaught stood in the parking lot in front of the main administrative building to listen to Pennsylvania Governor Tom Ridge and Connaught's President, Dave Williams, talk about ways that the company had planned for growth.

Tom Ridge was shown on the local television news channel giving Williams a check for a million dollars. It was the first time the governor had come to visit the campus and the first time the Commonwealth had offered a grant from its new Opportunity Fund, a $25 million initiative designed to keep jobs in the state.

"This is a company that has resources to locate anywhere in the world," Ridge said. "We think the grant is a great investment in our community. Biotechnology holds amazing promise as the growth industry for the next century, and I want to make Pennsylvania a leader in that movement."[1]

The grant, the newscaster said, supported a $9 million expansion project at the Swiftwater-based vaccine producer that included new

---

[1]Jeff Widmer, *The Spirit of Swiftwater: 100 Years at the Pocono Labs* (Scranton: University of Scranton Press, 1998), p. 99.

personnel, training, equipment, and an 87,500 square foot addition to Building 45 . . . the same building Jane had worked in before being moved to the trailers. It would be called Building 50.

The funding would help ensure the retention of jobs and the creation of new ones in Swiftwater. Ridge's Administration has also approved a $1million low-interest loan from the Pennsylvania Industrial Development Authority to help fund the company's capital investment program over the next five years, it was reported.[2]

Ridge was seen meeting with senior management, touring the facilities and then helping to conduct an experiment involving a test that detected antibody binding interactions. Then the cameras showed employees eating a picnic under tents that had been pitched outside for the occasion.

"I can't believe I'm not there, that I'm not part of this," Jane said to John that night after dinner. "It feels like I am getting fired all over again."

Patrick assigned his associate, Allen Tullar, to investigate The Americans with Disabilities Act (ADA), passed in 1990, which became effective four years earlier in 1992, to see if there were grounds to initiate a lawsuit. The law intended to eliminate illegal discrimination against those with disabilities. If they could prove that Jane had been discriminated against because of her Multiple Sclerosis, they had a case, but the law was so new that it was also uncharted territory.

"Title I prohibits employers, including cities and towns, from discriminating against qualified job applicants and workers who are or who become disabled. The law covers all aspects of employment including the application process and hiring, training, compensation, advancement, and any other employment term, condition, or privilege," Allen noted. "We'll need to prove that Jane is disabled as defined in the Act, that she was qualified for her job and could perform her duties with or without reasonable accommodation, and that her termination was based in part on her disability."

"The problem we will have is that it's a difficult law to interpret."

---

[2]Ibid, p. 99.

"Yea, but because it's so new, maybe that'll work for us." Allen was of medium build and height with a thin upper lip. His hair was receding but still brunette even though he teetered on forty. The only sign of aging, besides the hair, was the bags that had been forming under his eyes. He looked more like a middle school teacher than an attorney, but he was as approachable as a teacher, which worked in his favor.

Patrick nodded. Was he up for the challenge? He knew a lot of factors go into deciding whether or not to accept a new client, the principal one being, *will the ends justify the means?* Jane was likable; she seemed to have the support of her husband; that was critical to any case. He knew that sometimes lawyers ended up being counselors in more than law—sometimes they were therapists trying to right the wrong and helping clients endure the long judicial process. An intact support system made a difference to the outcome and to the process in getting there.

"The way Jane tells it, Connaught definitely demonstrated a lack of sensitivity in dealing with her," Patrick said to Allen.

"We both know there are two sides of the story. And we both know that corporations are notorious for their insensitivity. Throw-away employees and such. Nothing new there."

"But if what Jane said is true, and I found her to be honest and credible, she has clearly been subjected to discrimination. But taking on a pharmaceutical company with unlimited funds to defend isn't going to be easy."

"Since when did you need easy as a requirement?"

Patrick decided to take the case after deliberating about it for two weeks. He called Jane. "This will be an uphill battle, you realize, don't you?"

She didn't hesitate: "I'm up for the fight."

"It'll be the fight of your life. Your entire life will be examined from every angle and you will, like every client, most likely come to the moment when you will ask yourself if it's worth it all."

"Patrick, I am up for the challenge. I've been a fighter all my life, and this is my fight to win."

"The first thing we have to do is file a claim with the Pennsylvania Human Relations Commission. I need you to come in next week so we can sit down and get all the facts."

"You name the time. I'm spending most of my days looking for another job."

"Jane," Patrick paused. "Every case is built on facts, not emotions. Save them for the jury."

Patrick filed the claim. The Pennsylvania Human Relations Commission (PHRC) took months to respond. Jane called over the next few weeks that turned into months. Patrick reassured her that the length of time meant nothing; she was just one of hundreds of claims that a limited number of case workers and investigators had to review. Connaught would have to answer the claim and then the fact-finding conference would be scheduled.

Six months after the claim was filed with the Commission, Patrick received a response to the claim from Connaught.

"If Jane was this bad of an employee, I wouldn't have kept her either," Patrick said to Allen as he handed him the document.

"Typical defense strategy, not one positive statement. I guess we shouldn't have expected anything less."

"Arrogance drips from these pages—this might work in our favor. The Commission will pick up on this and maybe it will encourage them to further investigate the claim. I'll call Jane and tell her what they said, see how she responds. Based on her reaction, we should have some idea of how she would hold up in court."

Patrick called Jane later that afternoon and he read her the allegations Connaught was making against her.

"Those fuckers! After all I did for that company? I gave my life to them, and this is how they are going to portray me? Those sons-of-bitches. What're we going to do?"

"We'll see how the Commission responds. I'm sure they will be as turned off as we are. Arrogance always costs." Patrick hung up the receiver. He knew then and there that they had a winnable case, and he wanted nothing more than to expose the company for what they were and what they did—toss employees aside like a piece of malfunctioning equipment.

CHAPTER TWENTY

"Go Get 'Em"

Almost a year after Jane first consulted with Patrick, the PHRC, whose sole task was to enforce the state's anti-discrimination laws and promote equal opportunity, finally responded. The PHRC invited Gagliardo and legal counsel, along with Judy Stout and Connaught's legal representation, to their office in Harrisburg to present their case.

In preparation for the face-to-face meeting, Patrick tasked Jane with gathering evidence of all the positive things she had done for Connaught. Corporations had no memory of their own. They were like hard drives infected with a virus that lost whatever didn't work for them. Nothing new, he had seen it before, more times than he wanted to acknowledge, he told her.

Something about big corporations, and trillion dollar industries— they became entities, gods, a collective conscious without conscience.

Jane arrived at Patrick's office a week before the meeting with PHRC, lugging letters from the President of Connaught thanking her for her efforts on various projects, letters from customers commending her on her professionalism, patience and commitment, and even a nomination for the company award, "You Make a Difference."

"These are exactly what we are looking for to refute their position that you caused the company to lose thousands of dollars. I guess they forgot about the millions you saved them in starting the in-house tele-marketing department, on top of everything else."

"Now you know why I feel that I've been unjustly fired. Pat, I worked really hard for them. I loved my job. Do you understand?" She tilted her head as she spoke to him, sitting across from his desk.

"Maybe the company ought to have a new theme song—'What have you done for me lately,' might be a good choice."

She laughed, but the laughter opened the way for tears to flow. "I'm sorry."

Patrick pointed to the tissue box.

"I don't know what it is, but when I laugh I start to cry."

Patrick waited a moment before he told Jane they needed to discuss something before going to conference. "What is it that you want from Connaught? Under the law, you could be entitled to a return to employment with them, your wages and benefits from the time you were fired to today, and into the future, and damages for the emotional trauma they have caused you. What do you want?"

"What I want is for them to apologize. I want them to admit they were wrong." Jane looked at him as if for emphasis. "That is what I want more than anything."

"Even if we win, you will never get an apology. Their arrogance runs deep—deeper than any of us are ever going to want to recognize. Companies like Connaught don't ever admit to making a mistake. You aren't wrestling with a person, even if that person is Judy Stout, or Chris Kirby. You are wrestling with an entity that has arms and legs that stretch across the world. A heck of an opponent, I can assure you."

"I can tell you right now I could never work for them again. How do I know they wouldn't do the same thing to me somewhere down the road? John and I are suffering financially. I got a job working as a telemarketer, but I'm not making anywhere near what I did with Connaught, and we have no benefits. John is killing himself, working harder than ever before, and we've had to struggle to find money to put the boys through college." Jane lowered her head, and in a faint voice said, "I am so ashamed."

"The only thing you might get out of them is monetary compensation. It's like a divorce—it's all about the money."

"It is. It really is like a divorce, at least for me."

"That's one way of putting it. But you have to come up with some demand, some payment for the discrimination."

"We have to come up with a figure?"

"Yea, at least as a starting point."

"How much should we ask? How much could we win?"

"I wish I knew, but there's no book I can turn to or formula to use in situations like this. We'll go to the conference and see what they have to offer. Whatever the amount, it will never be enough or what you deserve, but it's better than where you are now."

"Seems like anywhere is better than where we are now." Jane blew her nose. "I'm sorry, it's just so upsetting."

Jane dressed in one of the suits she had bought for Connaught, a coffee-colored jacket and matching skirt. A red blouse beneath—it would serve as a reminder that she had to be fire herself. In the mirror, the short, stocky, 44-year-old woman seemed like an impostor of herself. Donning the suit reminded her of who she had once thought herself to be. *Had she really let a fuckin' company do that to her?*

Women's magazines—they talked about sexual harassment, sexism, that kind of discrimination; being female was the only disability they addressed for the most part. She remembered the first interview she had at Connaught—how she had consulted all the latest women's magazines on what to wear, how to dress for success. What would the title of the article be now: "How to Dress for Discrimination," or "How to Dress for Vengeance," or something ludicrous . . . ? The scent of Jessica McClintock cologne still clung to the polyester fabric, the cologne she had worn everyday to counteract the smell of burning eggs.

Somehow her reflection mirrored nothing but ridicule and mockery. *Told you you were too stupid to amount to anything . . . women are good for one thing—cooking, making babies, and satisfying their husbands. They didn't belong in any boardroom, they belonged in the bedroom, and the more women in the workplace, the more the boardroom turned into a bedroom; it was her father's words, but her voice.*

When John walked into the bedroom, he said, "You look great, Babe."

"Liar."

"Don't let them do it to you over and over again. They win every time."

"I'm a wreck about today."

"I'll be with you every step of the way."

Harrisburg rose from the Pennsylvania farm fields like gray stalks of corn. Some buildings looked tired. Other new skyscrapers dominated the cityscape, mighty-looking against the industrial gray on that cool, cloudy spring day. To the north were the Appalachian Mountains. The Susquehanna River cut through the capital. Jane opened the car window to breathe in the river-drenched air. The multiple bridges, with their curved bases, one alongside the other, gave a classical sense of order and architectural rhythm to the place.

The PHRC was located in a strip mall in a not-so-desirable neighborhood. Decay, ruin, and hopelessness were written in the air like invisible graffiti. They stepped inside the waiting room that was small with a few mismatched chairs and a side table with outdated magazines. The walls, a dingy avocado green. Patrick was waiting there, wearing a gray pin-striped suit, white shirt and navy tie. He stood when Jane and John entered.

"It's good that we don't have to share the room with anyone from Connaught," Patrick said. "Jane, prepare yourself. This will be grueling—good practice for court, if we get that far. This is going to be harder than you think, more emotionally draining than you can imagine."

"I'm stronger than you think, stronger than you can imagine."

"She is," John said, smiling.

"I'm afraid, John, you'll have to wait here. They won't let you into the conference room."

A few minutes later, a woman behind a desk in front of them stood up and requested they follow her. She was Latino—young, good-looking, wearing a tight skirt. Jane couldn't help but focus on the sway of her hips. Her name was Alma, she informed them, and she led them to a spartan but functional conference room. No one could accuse the state of spending too much money on this department.

A middle-aged African-American woman greeted them, introducing herself as Gayle, their case worker.

Patrick leaned over to Jane. "This is good—she's a woman and she knows all about prejudice—we may have just found someone who is sympathetic to us. Keep your fingers crossed."

Jane pulled a worn-thin upholstered chair out from beneath the table. Her stockings swished against each other as she sat down; it seemed like the only noise in the oxygen-deprived room.

A moment later, Judy Stout and two men appeared in the room as if they had been hiding in the shadows somewhere.

Jane's hands trembled. She hid them under the table. Her legs started to twitch; she spread them so that they did not rub against each other and swish, swish, swish throughout the entire meeting.

"Carl Greco," the man in the three-piece shiny suit said, as he reached out his hand toward Patrick.

Patrick extended his hand, "Patrick Reilly."

What did it feel like, shaking hands with the enemy? This was her fight, her case, not Patrick's, Jane reminded herself, refusing to extend her hand to him. She knew the name Greco. He had been Judy's boss before Judy had become Jane's boss, when shifting from the legal department to the customer service department. It was also his name that was on the letter Judy had sent Jane in response to demanding her rental deposit back, years ago.

Judy wore a dark gray pantsuit with black heels. Of course, Jane thought, Judy knew better.

"Hello, Jane," Judy said, as if to intimidate Jane, standing over and above her.

Jane's spine turned into a steel rod. *Stare her in the face. Stand up for yourself, no matter how tall they appear.*

It was as if Patrick read her body and nodded in approval.

Gayle interrupted: "Let's get started, shall we?"

Reilly could only advise Jane, as Greco did Stout. In the end, Connaught maintained their stance that Jane was mistake prone, had cost them a bundle of money, and was a detriment to the company, so they had no choice but to fire her. No apology, of course, as expected.

Letters of recommendation from the President, colleagues, and consumers alike made no difference, not even the award she had been nominated for, according to Stout, Greco and the legal assistant, who did little other than lean over and whisper something in Greco's ear on occasion.

"Connaught should consider making an offer to settle," the case worker said. "I think Ms. Gagliardo has a plausible claim."

They offered about ten thousand dollars, the same offered Jane on the day she was fired. Patrick smirked as if he had just heard a bad joke.

"This is an insult," Patrick said to the case worker.

Like a choreographed dance, Greco, Stout and assistant stood up, pushing their chairs out but not back into place, and left the conference room.

Patrick motioned to Jane that it was time to go as well. All that was going to be said was said; the lean offer was on the table and would remain there. Jane stood up and reached out her hand to Gayle.

"Thank you so much for your time."

Gayle shook her hand, closed her folder and stood to leave. "You'll be hearing from me."

Down the hall, Jane imagined herself a prisoner who had just been sentenced, the beginning of the end. John stood when they entered the waiting room and followed the silent train out to the parking lot.

"What do you think?" Jane asked Patrick out in the parking lot.

"I think they're arrogant assholes! But I got a good feeling from the case worker. I think she believes you were wronged. Unfortunately, she doesn't have the authority to order that Connaught do anything to compensate you, and I don't think there's enough based on your case alone for a referral to the Attorney General to file an action against Connaught."

"So what do we do next?" John asked.

"We wait for her decision."

"How long will that take? This whole process is so time consuming," Jane said.

"I know. But there's no real time limit. We've waited this long for a conference, we can wait for her decision. Once we receive that decision, then we can file a complaint in Federal court against Connaught, and the real battle will begin."

"The battle's been real for me for a long time already."

"You just have to be patient. There's nothing slower than our justice system. Nothing, I am convinced."

Four months later a letter came from the PHRC. The case worker had found evidence of discrimination, but not enough for the Commonwealth of Pennsylvania to get involved. A form letter had come granting Gagliardo the "Right to Sue," the prerequisite for starting the lawsuit, with one exception. Handwritten on the bottom of the letter were the words, "Go get 'em, counselor!" Those four words were the inspiration for the next four years.

CHAPTER TWENTY-ONE

The Road Less Traveled

Without a doubt, trials take conviction. Conviction Reilly had, and a good measure of realism. Since the Disabilities Act was so new, it upped the ante, but in which direction?

After receiving PHRC's right-to-sue letter, he had ninety days to file suit. During that period, he and Tullar researched the Americans with Disabilities Act (ADA) itself and the few cases interpreting it. By deadline, Reilly filed a claim based both upon the ADA and the Pennsylvania Human Relations Act since the state of Pennsylvania act has no limitations on the amount of damages, while the ADA had a limit of $300k based on the number of employees at Connaught. A notice came that the suit had been assigned to a judge. Now came the fun part—the preparation for trial, the squirm, the game, the interplay between plaintiff and defendant. Connaught was a worthy opponent.

Reilly had learned early on in his practice that justice is supposed to be about righting a wrong, but it rarely worked that way. There's never a way to go back, to return to what was, to change history. Award money is the only way to transform the future, to redeem it, at least in this case. But Greco knew, as all lawyers know, that proving injury, proving damages and trying to recover them was a long shot.

Sometimes arrogance was a self-fulfilling prophecy, or so it seemed. Surely Jane knew the world suffered a deep coldness . . . surely she knew.

A magistrate judge had been assigned to work out the possibility of a settlement between Jane and Connaught. Connaught offered $50,000. Patrick insisted it wasn't a reasonable offer, but he was willing to come to the bargaining table.

"If you go to court, Jane, you could end up with nothing, nothing except my bill."

"I'll take my chances."

"Listen, it's an offer; it's a start. I have dozens of discrimination cases that have never settled, some that appear an easy win."

"I think we ought to consider settling," John, sitting next to her in the office, chimed in.

"What the hell? You two are going to decide for me; you're going to tell me to accept an offer!"

"Try to take the emotion out of it," Patrick said.

"Really? You try to take the emotion out of it. You aren't risking a fuckin' penny to do this, so it's easy for you." Jane felt her face redden. She wanted to say more. Her tongue twisted and curled inside her salivating mouth.

"Calm down, Jane," John said.

"This isn't about us, John. It's about me. Neither one of you has the passion for this. I wonder if you'd feel different if it was you who had been wronged. I've got to go." She stood up, grabbed her purse, turned away from Patrick and John and moved toward the door.

"Jane," Patrick said, trying to stop her. "You have to look at the whole picture."

"No, you have to look at me. I have this burning inside me. I have to finish this fight, and I will, with or without either one of you. You can both bow out, but I am in for the long haul, no matter what."

John stood up, following Jane out of the office, turning to Patrick: "We'll call."

"Listen, maybe you ought to settle, not for $50,000 but for a more reasonable amount and consider it retribution, Babe."

"Don't Babe me, not now. I get it that you aren't as passionate as I am. But I am not going to fold—not for you. Forget your Italian ass!"

"Patrick knows his business. If he didn't think he can get them to make a good offer offer, he wouldn't tell you to take it."

"Ok, so for the last four fuckin' years, while we're both working our asses off between our four jobs, we should just say, ok? You son of a bitch, and that son of a bitch lawyer—it didn't happen to you. You don't care. I know, I know without a doubt, if a jury heard my story they would side with me. I know it."

"We could really use the money now. We have college tuition to think about!"

"Listen to me, I know the money has been tight. Do you really think I want to clean motel rooms on the weekends and sell time shares during the week? You don't think that every fuckin' day I think about my job at Connaught and long for it back? You don't think that I wrestle every day with the fact that I have this fuckin' diagnosis and I ask myself, what will I lose next? You don't think that my job was just about money, do you? I thought you knew me better than that!" Her voice cracked and reached a crescendo before she started coughing. "You both want to take the easy way out—well, there is no easy way out."

"What the hell, Jane. You've got such a sense of justice that you're going to risk our future to be right? So what if a jury doesn't empathize with you, then what? We are into Patrick for thousands and thousands of dollars—just so you can be fuckin' right?"

"Fuck you."

"Fuck you back."

Before John left for his second job selling cars that evening, Jane cooked a pasta dinner—a necessary prerequisite for John, even though she added a little spit to it. Nothing he liked better than spaghetti. Jane watched him eat it, noodle by noodle, sucking it down his mouth and disappearing. His coloring was beginning to fade. Was it just age? Was it the stress of their lives? Should she give in?

"Listen, I'm sorry, but I just can't do this. I can't let the company get away with it. They'll end up doing it again and again."

"Really, do you think they will change even if you go to court and win? Do you really think they will change?"

"I don't care if I win one dollar. We wouldn't have to pay Patrick, who I'd like to fire right about now. I have to tell the story. I have stood alone in the past, and I can stand alone now."

She watched as he left for work, saying nothing more. But there on his plate was a small portion of uneaten food, something he had never left behind before. His hulking mass, his shoulders, his strong legs . . . the cigarette smell on his clothes wafted behind him. Fuck him.

Later that night, unable to sleep, Jane went downstairs to the dining room table and wrote Reilly a letter.

Dear Mr. Reilly,

Today I was very disappointed in the way the call with Connaught went. But more so I was very disappointed in the fact that you no longer believe in this case. I know that you have case laws that you know to be facts, but how do you think those laws became that way?

There was a client and a lawyer that fought to make sure that those injustices never happen again. Well, I believe that we also will make a case law that other lawyers and clients can use.

I was fired unjustly and I had taken from me a job that I loved and I know I could have done well if Connaught had just taken the extra work away. But Judy fired me because she was uncomfortable with my MS and she stated so in front of witnesses.

I know and believe from the very bottom of my soul that I have been violated and discriminated against because of my MS. I know that this injustice must be stopped.

I also know that if you do not have the same passion and fight for this case as I do, then I need to know that as well. We have to be on the same page, we have to think the same way or they will win.

I know that if lay men/women just like me were to hear this story they would also know the injustice that has been done to me. I have this burning in my stomach and heart that tells me to fight this. How many more are there like me out there that other companies are doing this to? How many others are willing to fight for what is right and true?

I know I am only one and please don't make me stand alone in this. You must have the fight and the passion for this.

If you don't then please bow out and let me find someone that does. I feel that you are the one to make sure that justice is served and I also feel that you can make this happen. So please stop telling me about all of the cases that didn't make it and focus on this one that will. Please trust me. I know I am not wrong about this.

My husband is not in agreement with me to send you this letter, but I feel you are a reasonable man and someone who wants to right a wrong, well here is your chance.

Sincerely,
Jane Gagliardo

A few days later Patrick pulled Jane's letter from the pile of mail on his desk. He knew it couldn't be good. Why else would she send a letter? They hadn't spoken since she left his office angry over his and John's attempt to convince her to settle with Connaught. Would anything satisfy her? He knew how the system worked, she didn't. Where was her reason? Justice always came with a dollar sign in front of it, didn't it?

Patrick looked out of the window at the steel-colored sky before tearing the envelope open. For a split second he remembered what it felt like to stand on a field soft with rain and thawing frost, and how the air stung his lungs. How different his life was now. No rhythm, no seasons, no rest, no fragrant earth, just stale office air. Unexpected harvests, yes, but losses too. His first wife had left him. He wanted to enter a plea of not guilty to the invisible courtroom in his head, to the judge that passed sentences on his life.

"I am not guilty of driving my wife away." He had said it over and over again until he believed it. Maybe it was just that the job was tough on relationships—too many hours, too many dramas. Home was the last place he wanted verdicts, even if he felt he had to justify the marriage itself for years.

In his head the song, *Come on Baby Light My Fire*, crescendoed. *You weren't supposed to leave my life in ashes*. He had custody of his two children. Sometimes, his body ached for them like his old football injury.

He opened the letter and read it, then stared out the window again, longing for the sounds of the land, the groans of trees, the moans of wind, rather than the phones ringing, the murmur of voices out in reception, the heaviness of feet on concrete, and disgruntled clients. He knew Jane had what he didn't. She was right—he didn't have the passion she had for her case. He didn't think it warranted it. Who was she? An everyday woman who had been fired. Who would care? Could she make others care? He hated to lose.

Unfolding Jane's letter he had tucked into his briefcase, he read it again. Was it worth going up against one of the most profitable industries in the world, and one of the most prestigious employers in Pennsylvania? Was it worth the professional risk? Would it break the hold of passivity on his life?

The only conviction he had ever wanted was the kind that slammed the bad guys behind bars, at least the bad guys he wasn't defending. Perhaps it was time to remember why he entered law in the first place, rather than push for easy wins and sure outcomes. Maybe he ought to go the distance, agree to run with the case all the way to trial, a case he was sure he couldn't win. He knew then that he suffered from a different kind of disability, the malaise of money, the non-living of the living, the sure thing over the unsure, all the symptoms of a disease for which he wasn't sure there was a cure.

CHAPTER TWENTY-TWO

The Trial

Jane borrowed her brother's camper since she and John couldn't afford to pay for a hotel room for however many nights they might have to stay for the trial. They arrived at the Harrisburg East Campground the day before the trial was scheduled to begin. Jane's brother had brought his camper up from south Jersey for them to use. He had already hooked up the water, piled firewood near the stone pit, and stocked the miniature refrigerator.

Inside, the tiny kitchen wasn't well suited for an Italian cook. The shower stall was large enough for only half of John's body. Somehow, though, it all seemed to fit into the scheme of things, this sense of displacement, of a place somewhat familiar and foreign at the same time, a place that seemed to squeeze the life out of them. Jane thought maybe it would come down to this one day, being forced to live in a trailer if she lost the case. The television screen was so small, John complained he had to wear his reading glasses to see it. His head skimmed the ceiling when he walked down the middle of the camper.

John started a fire while Jane unpacked their clothes, then filled a large pot with water and placed it over the grill to boil for pasta. The spaghetti sauce she had made at home warmed in another pot. Such a ritual far from home comforted her. They ate dinner on the fold-up table, watching for the sunset, and later retired to watch TV, trying with all their might not to think or talk about the trial.

The next morning, September 18, they rose early to cook their breakfast. John stirred the embers from the night before, added a few pieces of wood, while Jane wiggled a pot of coffee onto the center of the grill. The air was still and sweet with summer. Drawing a deep inhale, she reminded herself that life would be good again, that this too shall pass, and that they would survive no matter what. Somewhere in her gut she knew that if she could only tell her story the jury would understand. Her hands trembled as she pulled them away from the fire.

"This is it, John."

"Yep, this is it."

"What if I don't win?"

"All you have to be awarded is one dollar, and we won't have to pay Pat's fee. By the time the trial ends, we'll owe him over a hundred grand if we don't win. You have to win."

Jane shifted the pot over the highest flames. They were already in financial ruin with her job loss. Working as a telemarketer didn't help enough.

"John, you stuck by me when you thought I should have settled out of court. We fought too much during these last years. This fight isn't just for me, but for everyone who has a disability. What they did was wrong."

"You've always stood up for yourself. I know who you are, Jane. I may not have agreed with you. It's a risk, a huge risk. We'll manage somehow, even if we lose."

She stared into the fire, listening for the water to boil, glancing up to see John's hulking body folded into the chair, making them about the same height when she stood next to him. He had loved her, rescued her from her family as she did him, but he couldn't stand between her and the world now, or the things that haunted her body. But, he was all she could ask for. He was enough in this lifetime.

"Come on, I'll help you take a shower. The water's taking forever," she said as her feet shuffled across the grass and patch of bare earth.

John shed his clothes and ran the water until it was warm enough to stand under. Too large to fit and turn around in the stall, Jane held the shower hose to wash his back. They laughed at themselves. She wrapped a towel around him, remembering that morning on her thirtieth birthday when he helped her into the shower and dried her off.

The water boiled and hissed and spurted and percolated outside. While John dressed, she set the pot aside and slid an iron skillet over the now steady flames and cooked bacon and eggs, throwing a few slices of bread on top the grill.

They ate in silence, watching the sun rise over the river, leaving its bread crumbs of light. Afterwards, Jane showered and dressed in a pair of black slacks and a blue knit top. She grabbed her cane even though she told herself no matter what she would walk into the courtroom leaning on nothing and no one.

———

Pat arrived the night before the trial. He had strained his back over the weekend and he knew the drive alone would be excruciating. That evening he worked on his opening statement in the hotel room and memorized it until he was so saturated with words, he couldn't remember a word of it. He slept on the floor, hoping his herniated disk would slip back. Waking early, he ran the hot water in the tub, then eased down into the wet heat for a half hour, but found little relief. Everything inside him burned as he struggled to dress, gathered his material, and lugged it to his car. He wondered if Jane had felt this burning in her body everyday. Today, maybe this pain would make him a better lawyer.

This trial would be unprecedented territory—The Americans with Disability Act (ADA) was so new there was no way to predict the outcome or the jury's reaction to such a case. He suspected it was the trial of his career, never mind Jane's life.

The Ronald Reagan Federal Building, a monolith of glass, mirrored the cityscape and sky and clouds like a painting in motion. Jane couldn't breathe when she saw Pat waiting for her outside the building, a briefcase in hand, legal books under his arm. A tentative smile crossed his face. The same smile she had seen at other times—one she *interpreted* as an attempt to persuade, to offer hope, even when there was only a sliver's worth. Either way, he won; he and he alone, she thought.

"Are you ready for one of the biggest days of your life?" he asked her as she struggled to get out of the car.

"I'm ready for the truth to be told. I'm not ready for anything else." Her entire body tremored, and she couldn't discern whether it was nerves or the disease. "I can't stop shaking."

"Everyone feels that way when they are about to go to court."

"Thanks, Pat."

They waited for John to park the car and join them, and then endured the scrutiny of security. On the other side were elevators that would take them to Courtroom Number Four.

"Wheelchair coming through. Everyone move please. We have a woman in a wheelchair." The voice was harsh, demanding. A woman in a nurse's uniform barked through the crowd, pushing Chris Kirby, Connaught's token MS disabled employee. Kirby's presence reminded Jane of where she might one day end up. She was proof that Connaught honored their disabled employees, proof in living color that Jane's claim was unfounded. The nurse made such a spectacle of it all that it was difficult to feel compassion.

"Move aside, please, wheelchair coming through," the nurse cried out, again and again.

Jane, John and Pat moved aside.

"You've got to be kidding me—this is so obvious," Pat whispered to them. "Shameless."

Chris' gaze remained transfixed on the floor. Her tall and thin body appeared caved-in, as if she knew she were the main exhibit. A silent cry seemed to intrude the world of noise. She hid behind her curtain of dark blonde hair.

"She's embarrassed, you can see that. I feel sorry for her, that she has to be paraded around like this," Jane said.

Outside Courtroom Number Four, Pat said, "We've reached the point of no return. Once we enter that door, there is no exit. Once we enter that door we'll go all the way. There's no turning back, no negotiation."

"I really believe that if I can tell my story, the jurors will understand. I have to tell my story."

Pat nodded. He never said anything negative before stepping foot into a courtroom. Never.

Jane and Pat went inside while John stayed outside as instructed, pacing the hallway, waiting for his call to the witness stand, probably hours away. Inside the courtroom, Alan Tullar, Pat's associate, was setting up legal pads and files at the plaintiff's table on the left side of the courtroom, closest to the jury box. There was a comforting presence about him, Jane surmised, something sturdy and steadfast.

The room lacked the old dark wood theater of historic courtrooms—it was simple, bland, vanilla, with no architectural interest. The only dramas here were human, an architecture of flesh and bone, persuasion and argument, no echo, no sense of old voices having stained or deepened the hue of the wooden paneling. A lectern was positioned next to the jury box. To their right was the defendant's table. Carl Greco and associates entered with Kirby in tow.

"Remember what I told you, Jane. Every trial has its highs and lows. Carl is going to make you sound like a rotten person. Prepare yourself. Don't let what he says affect you because if you give in to it, it will affect your testimony and how you present yourself."

"My entire life has prepared me for this moment. I can stand up to any bully."

Before the trial began, the judge called the attorneys into chambers. She told Pat that she wanted Jane to be the first witness. Pat knew Jane wasn't ready to go first. She would be more nervous, unsure of herself, no matter how prepared she thought she was, but it wasn't up for discussion.

In early September, in this room, Judge Yvette Kane had encouraged Jane to settle out of court when they had gathered at the courthouse for jury selection. A $200,000 offer was discussed. Jane refused. The judge unzipped her robe then and draped it over her desk chair. She sat on the edge of the mahogany desk and spoke to Jane as if she were a friend, asking her about her family and life, and how a trial is never a sure thing, but a settlement is. After further discourse, Jane agreed. When the judge called Carl into chambers, he denied any offer had been settled on.

"We're going to trial," Judge Kane said. "Jane is a very credible witness."

Pat agreed—Jane would be called to the witness stand first. Then he, Judge Kane, and Carl entered the courtroom in single file.

Fourteen jurors, ranging in age from the late twenties to mid-fifties, were escorted into the jury box and sat down behind a wooden rail, nearest the lectern where the lawyers would stand. Jane made deliberate eye contact with each one as if to say, I am you. I am you.

She and Pat had chosen three jurors that were ex-military and one had been employed as an insurance adjuster before he had been eliminated from his job. Jane searched the pool for the guy who had showed up on that hot day in a Grateful Dead T-shirt. He wore it, they were sure, with the intention of not being picked. It turned out he was an ex-marine. She spotted him in the back row.

Judge Kane settled into her chair. She had a kind face. Her eyes turned downward a bit and her crow's feet gave her the appearance of a wise woman. Her upper lip was curve-less. She wore her brunette hair short and layered.

"Mr. Reilly, I recognize the plaintiff for opening statements." Her voice smooth, calming, and authoritative.

Patrick walked to the lectern. "Thank you. May it please the Court, counsel, ladies and gentlemen of the jury, again my name is Patrick Reilly and together with my co-counsel, Allen Tullar, I have the pleasure and responsibility of representing Jane Gagliardo in this action.

"What you're going to hear about over the next several days is a story of arrogance, apathy and indifference. You're going to hear the story of how a devoted and dedicated employee is treated in today's cold business world.

"This is an action which has been brought under the Americans with Disabilities Act and the Pennsylvania Human Relations Act. We're going to show to you that Jane Gagliardo was disabled. That she was able to do her job. That she was terminated from her job in part because of her disability. That she suffered damages as a result of this.

"How are we going to show you that Jane Gagliardo was disabled? Jane Gagliardo herself is going to tell you that she suffers from Multiple Sclerosis. You wouldn't know it by looking at her because from all outward appearances she appears to be a normal, healthy individual, but you will hear about her symptoms and how they affected her.

"One of those symptoms that you're going to hear about is fatigue and how it affected her at work, how it affected her ability to concentrate, her ability to focus and her ability to remember. It affected her memory.

"You'll hear that those symptoms were aggravated by stress and how stress made those symptoms even worse, and it affected in part her ability to do her job.

"Mrs. Gagliardo started with Connaught Laboratories in March of 1987. . . . You'll hear that at one point in time after working a shift at Connaught Laboratories she took a part-time job with a telemarketing firm in the Pocono area to learn the telemarketing business so that she could bring back the knowledge that she learned about that business to Connaught Laboratories, so that they could open a telemarketing business as part of their operation of their business, and she did that. She stayed in that position for a period of time before returning to the customer accounts department as a customer account representative.

"Until 1996 Jane Gagliardo received performance appraisals on a yearly basis that were in the commendable range, and as a result of that, she received yearly raises, and she also received a monetary performance award.

"You'll hear that although she was not perfect, we're not suggesting that she was a perfect worker, and you'll see that she did make mistakes, just as other customer service representatives, or CARs, made mistakes, but nevertheless she was an asset to Connaught Laboratories. You'll see that other CARs looked up to her, looked to her when they had questions about how to perform their job and what they needed to do, how to do certain things. They looked to her as a resource to help them whenever they needed any assistance.

"You'll see that there were various letters commending her for the service that she did in her personnel file for the things that she did over the years. You will hear that she worked overtime. You will hear that on one particular occasion she came in on Christmas Day to do part of her job because there was an emergency. She gave of her time.

"You'll hear that Jane was always looking for more to do at her place of employment because she was proud of what she did and she liked her job.

"For eight years 11 months, almost nine years, Jane Gagliardo had absolutely no involvement with the disciplinary process at Connaught

Laboratories. That all changed in 1996 when an individual named Judith Stout became her supervisor.

"You're going to hear that Judy Stout was a paralegal in the medical legal department and was in fact supervised by Mr. Greco, who is here on behalf of Connaught Laboratories today.

"You'll hear that Miss Stout's appraisals, her performance appraisals, were not commendable. You will hear that she had difficulty getting along with others, that she was not a team player, that she did not finish projects at all, and if she did finish them, they were not finished on time. And her rating under the Connaught Laboratory performance appraisals was not commendable, but you'll hear it required coaching, and that was a category that you'll see is in their performance appraisals.

"Despite the fact that she received these types of ratings, in 1994 Judith Stout was promoted to a supervisor in the customer account management department, and in 1996 she became Jane Gagliardo's supervisor.

"Within one month after becoming Mrs. Gagliardo's supervisor, she issued a verbal warning to Mrs. Gagliardo for some mistakes that had been made. You'll hear that this is the first step in the disciplinary process at Connaught Laboratories.

"The mistakes that Mrs. Gagliardo made were related, you'll hear, to new programs that Connaught had implemented, and you'll hear about something called Biological Ordering Agreement or Biological Ordering Program and a program called doctor outbound calls. Those were relatively new programs, and you'll hear what was involved in those. And you'll hear Mrs. Gagliardo admit that she had difficulty with these particular programs early on.

"You'll also hear that at the time that Miss Stout provided the oral warning to Mrs. Gagliardo, she was aware that Mrs. Gagliardo had Multiple Sclerosis.

"Mrs. Gagliardo was diagnosed in 1989 approximately and when she found out about it, she told her supervisor. When she moved back into the customer account department, she told her supervisor that she had Multiple Sclerosis. There are numerous documents in her personnel file at Connaught Laboratories, making reference to her Multiple Sclerosis, including a document from her physician indicating that she had it, in response to a request for an accommodation in 1995 or 1996.

"And you'll hear that certain accommodations had been made for Mrs. Gagliardo. . . . In one instance her desk was raised up so that she would have her arms at a different level for her to perform her work. And in another particular instance you'll hear that the heat in the trailer that she was working in was adjusted because of her Multiple Sclerosis.

"You're going to hear that Miss Stout came to Jane Gagliardo at some point in early 1996 and asked her for information on Multiple Sclerosis, but you'll learn that that information was provided to Miss Stout and instead of opening it and looking at it, she stuck it in her desk drawer and never opened it."

Jane couldn't stop shuddering. She didn't feel her tears fall until they landed on her hands that were attempting to steady themselves by pressing them flat against the table. The jurors followed Pat's words as if he were writing them on the air. Can they know what it felt like to fade away into invisibility that MS caused her? No one wanted to see. Judy didn't want to see, didn't want to know. No one wanted to acknowledge the frailty of body or the diminishment of disease.

"Most of the customer account representatives had special projects that they performed as part of their normal responsibilities. These special projects were to take approximately 5 to 10 percent of their time. They were to perform these special projects in between doing their other duties, most importantly taking inbound calls, which they took the greater portion of the day, they were to take calls from customers, and they were to perform their special projects in between when they had time to do it.

"You'll hear that Mrs. Gagliardo volunteered to take the military account ordering and collections position, that it was one of the most demanding special projects that there was in the customer account representative or the customer account management department. She had the responsibility for that special project about one year, before Miss Stout became her supervisor. And you'll hear that it took about two hours a day of her time to perform that special project.

"Now Mrs. Gagliardo had told her prior supervisor, an individual named Wayne Neveling, that she felt the military project was taking too much of her time, was affecting her ability to do her job, and she asked that the responsibility be, if not in whole, at least in part be taken away from her.

"She also discussed this with Miss Stout when Miss Stout became her supervisor, particularly during this meeting in February of 1996 when she was given the first oral warning. It was discussed several times after that prior to the time that Mrs. Gagliardo was terminated, and you'll hear that it was never fully taken away from her. You'll hear that this would have been a reasonable accommodation to Jane Gagliardo.

"Following this initial meeting in February of 1996 when the oral warning was given, Miss Stout provided Miss Gagliardo with videotapes and audiotapes, and she told her that these were to assist her with her memory and her concentration because of the problems that she was having with her MS. And you'll hear that she asked her several times after this whether she watched the videotapes to help her with her memory and concentration.

"Less than one month after the oral warning a written caution is provided, and you'll hear that not one mistake which is mentioned in the written caution occurred after the oral warning was provided. Everything had occurred beforehand. Nothing occurred within that one month period, yet she was provided with a written warning.

"At that time Mrs. Gagliardo again asked for relief from the military ordering collection responsibility, and it still didn't happen."

Expose them . . . these were the words that repeated in Jane's head. Make sure they don't do this to anyone else, ever again.

"One month later, one more problem, one more mistake, she's placed on probation. This is the last step you'll see in the Connaught Laboratories policies and procedures before termination.

"Now you're also going to hear that Christine Kirby . . . " Pat pointed to Chris, slumped in her chair at the council table . . . "she participated in some of these meetings between Judith Stout and Jane Gagliardo. What is more important, you're going to hear about a meeting that occurred between Christine Kirby and Jane Gagliardo at some point in 1996 where Miss Kirby point blank asked Mrs. Gagliardo is your Multiple Sclerosis causing these problems, and Jane Gagliardo said yes.

"Miss Kirby was in the human relations department, responsible for Jane Gagliardo's department at Connaught Laboratories. It was her responsibility, you'll hear, to do something in response to that, and she did absolutely nothing.

"Finally, one more mistake was made on May 29, 1996. Mrs. Gagliardo was fired by Connaught Laboratories. You'll hear about the meeting that took place at that time in which Mrs. Gagliardo was present, Miss Kirby was present and Miss Stout was present.

"And you'll hear that she was presented with a confidentiality agreement to sign. She was asked to sign that and told that she would be paid a sum of money if that agreement was signed. You'll hear that a pen was placed in her hand, and she was asked to sign that. And when she didn't sign it, she was told if you'll just sign this, you'll make everyone else's life easier.

"You're then going to hear about the effect this had on Mrs. Gagliardo's life and the types of damages she suffered as a result of this, the embarrassment, the humiliation, being fired from a job that she loved and had been devoted to. You will hear about the fact that she had a son in college then, that she was worried about what she was going to tell her friends and family about what happened. You're going to hear about the lost wages that she suffered as a result of it, and you're going to hear about her emotional injuries. No one can or will be able to tell you what dollar figure should be placed on those emotional injuries. That will be your responsibility. And you'll also hear that there is a claim for punitive damages.

"Ladies and gentlemen, we're not going to present to you a perfect case because nothing is perfect in an imperfect world. But what we are going to do is show you by a preponderance of the evidence, utilizing both direct evidence and circumstantial evidence, that Jane Gagliardo was disabled, that she could do her job, that she was fired in part because of her disability and that she suffered damages as a result of that. We're going to show you that she had a legally protected right to her job, and that was violated. We're going to show you arrogance, apathy and indifference, and at the end we're going to ask you to consider all of that evidence and enter a verdict in favor of Jane Gagliardo.

"On behalf of Mrs. Gagliardo, I'd like to thank you in advance for your attention to this proceeding. Thank you."

Jane turned her head to see if she could spot John in the hallway, but there was no window. When Pat finished, the air felt cleansed, like after a rainstorm.

CHAPTER TWENTY-THREE

Connaught's Defense

Greco's Opening Statements

"Thank you, Mr. Reilly. Mr. Greco."

Greco stood, the chair scraped the floor. He sucked in and buttoned his jacket. His hair reflected the overhead lights as he sauntered to the lectern.

He had her in his hands. He wanted to reshape her. His words would crush her until she was created in the image he desired.

"May it please the Court, thank you, Your Honor. Counsel. Good morning, ladies and gentlemen. I'm Carl Greco, and I represent Connaught Labs, the defendant in this case. Now Judge Kane has mentioned to you about what the opening statement is all about, and at the time of the opening statement it's like a preview for a movie. And what the plaintiff has told you, as Judge Kane has mentioned, and what I am going to tell you now is not evidence. The plaintiff has the burden of proof and will have to prove Mrs. Gagliardo's claim in accordance with the law as told to you by Judge Kane.

"Let me tell you a little bit about my case. First of all, ladies and gentlemen, let me make it perfectly clear, Connaught Labs disputes Mrs. Gagliardo's claim. Our evidence and our witnesses and a lot more of the evidence and the witnesses in this case are going to show you that Mrs. Gagliardo wasn't terminated for anything related to Multiple Sclerosis. She was terminated because she made mistakes. Now termination is never easy, but in the interest of business it has to be done. And the evidence in this case will show you that it was done without any reliance whatsoever or any consideration whatsoever of her disability.

"Connaught Laboratories manufactures vaccines. They are a healthcare company, and they manufacture vaccines for influenza, whooping cough vaccine that's administered primarily to children, polio vaccines, and they also manufacture vaccines for a little more exotic type diseases like typhoid fever, yellow fever, travelers' vaccines. And they sell these vaccines to their customers, and their customers are physicians, pharmacists and others in the healthcare profession who use those vaccines in the fight against disease."

What about the disease of deception? What about the disease of discrimination? What about these—the questions screamed in Jane's head. She studied the jurors—they appear bored, almost, as if Greco was lecturing more than engaging them. He was like a bad actor.

"Now the evidence in this case is going to show you what—how Connaught sells their product. There are sales people out in the field who call on customers and provide information about products, but for many of the customers of the company the only contact they have with the company or a significant contact they have with the company is the Customer Account Representatives, the person inside, the person who takes the order, the person who has to arrange for shipping of the order and the person who provides them information about their relationship with Connaught. And you're going to hear the evidence in this case and the witnesses tell you how important a position it is."

That's right . . . how important a position it is. It was. The whole world seemed crowded in here, listening to him, listening to him make her sound like an idiot. What was on trial here is so much more than discrimination . . . her integrity, her character, her life was on trial.

"And you're going to hear from Judith Stout. Judith is a long term employee at Connaught, and Mrs. Stout is a manager in the customer account management department, and she was Mrs. Gagliardo's supervisor at the time she was terminated. Now Mrs. Stout is going to tell you about the mistakes that Mrs. Gagliardo was making, how she learned of those mistakes, the discussions she had and what she did.

"You're going to hear from Rosemary Kindrew. Now Rosemary Kindrew is not a supervisor, but she is a customer account management analyst, and she's going to tell you about the mistakes that Mrs. Gagliardo made and how she sat with Mrs. Gagliardo to help her and observe her in doing her job. And you're going to hear from Grace Cooper. Now Grace Cooper is the head of customer account management. Grace Cooper is also a long term employee at Connaught. She knew Jane Gagliardo, Mrs. Gagliardo, very well, and she knew the job, and she knew what Mrs. Gagliardo was supposed to do and what she didn't do. And she's going to tell you about the mistakes that Mrs. Gagliardo made, about the process that they went through with her and about how she was finally terminated.

"Now when we were together on September 5 and when you were selected to sit on the jury in this case, I mentioned to you at that time that this case involved Multiple Sclerosis and issues regarding Multiple Sclerosis. You've heard the plaintiff's lawyer refer to that in his opening, and you're going to hear a lot in the course of this case about Multiple Sclerosis. And you're going to hear evidence that will be offered about the plaintiff's Multiple Sclerosis and its affect on her job. One of the witnesses that the plaintiff may call in this case is Dr. Peter Barbour. Dr. Barbour is Mrs. Gagliardo's treating physician for her Multiple Sclerosis. I want you to pay close attention to Dr. Barbour's testimony when he talks about his diagnosis and the care that he's prescribed for Mrs. Gagliardo and her Multiple Sclerosis.

"I have a little bit of an idea of what Dr. Barbour is going to say because I have had an opportunity before this trial to take his deposition. For those of you who may not know, a deposition is an opportunity for the lawyers to ask the parties in a case or the witnesses questions about their knowledge and about what they have done with respect to this particular case. And I took Dr. Barbour's deposition, and I expect that his testimony at this trial is going to be consistent with the way he testified when I deposed him and the way that he has expressed himself in his reports which will also be some of the documentary evidence that will be introduced at trial."

He acts as if he was smarter than everyone else in the courtroom. His posture was over-exaggerated and he tipped his nose toward the ceiling.

"In fact, ladies and gentlemen, many of the witnesses you're going to hear from have been deposed. I had a chance to take Mrs. Gagliardo's deposition in April of 1998. She was present, her lawyer was present before a court stenographer, and I had a chance to ask her questions about her job, about what she was doing, about her Multiple Sclerosis. And I expect that her testimony is going to be exactly as it was at the time I deposed her."

Pat leaned over to Jane, "He's just told them nothing."

"And I have prepared an enlargement for you of a snippet from her deposition. And I asked her—you can see, ladies and gentlemen, that the snippet indicates that it was taken from her transcript of her deposition on April 22. And I asked her: 'Okay. Did Multiple Sclerosis prevent you from doing your job?' And she answered in her deposition under oath at that time: 'No.'"

Again, Pat tilted his head toward Jane's ear—"He still doesn't get it. He doesn't understand The Americans with Disabilities Act," and then he shook his head.

"Now you're going to hear testimony about the errors that she made. You're going to hear testimony about the importance of the customer account representatives, and you're going to hear testimony about Multiple Sclerosis. But all of this testimony, ladies and gentlemen, is going to show you that Mrs. Gagliardo is not disabled, that she made mistakes, and that she was properly terminated. Now at the end of the case after all the evidence I'm going to have a chance to come back to you and ask you at that time and argue to you at that time that you should render your verdict in accordance with the evidence that you have heard, the evidence that's going to show you today that Mrs. Gagliardo was not disabled, that she made mistakes and that she was properly terminated. . . ."

"Thank you, Mr. Greco." Judge Kane said.

Opening statements . . . what they do is open you up to order and chaos all at the same time, to truth and deception, to angels and demons that are fighting inside the courtroom. The jurors' eyes followed Greco back to the table.

Jane smelled his sickly sweet cologne mixed with a tinge of sweat as he unbuttoned his jacket before sitting down.

"Mr. Reilly, your first witness."

"Plaintiff calls Jane Gagliardo," Pat said.

Jane fought to stand up without wincing. Her right leg dragged as she moved toward the chair. Pat began his direct examination, asking her where she lived, how long she'd lived in East Stroudsburg, how long she'd been married.

"Thirty years in April."

"In 1995 and 1996 did anyone else reside with you?"

"Yes, my son John and my son Anthony."

"How many children do you have?"

"I have three sons."

"And could you give us their names and ages, please?"

"Joseph will be 29, John will be 25 and Anthony is 22."

"And where are they all now?"

"Joseph lives with his wife in San Antonio, Texas. John is stationed in North Carolina, Fort Bragg, and Anthony lives in Parsippany, New Jersey."

"How old are you?

"I'm 47."

"In 1996 how old were you?"

Her voice cracked. "I'm sorry, I'm very nervous."

"These are supposed to be the easy questions, Mrs. Gagliardo."

"I know. Forty-four, forty-five."

"Okay. What is your educational background?"

"High school education."

"Did you attend any post high school institutions?"

"No."

"When did you become employed by Connaught Laboratories?"

"March of 1987."

"What kind of work generally did you do prior to that time?"

"I worked for a bank for eight years."

"What did you do for the bank?"

"I worked in administration. I did clerical work."

"Okay. You have Multiple Sclerosis. Correct?"

"Yes, sir."

"When were you first diagnosed with Multiple Sclerosis?"

"It was suspected at the age of 30."

"Okay. When did it finally become diagnosed as being Multiple Sclerosis?"

"It was around 1992, '94, somewhere there."

"Were you employed by Connaught Laboratories when it was first suspected that you had Multiple Sclerosis?"

"No."

"Okay. What was it—what were the symptoms that you first experienced?"

"I was numb completely on my right."

"When you say completely on your right side, could you be more specific?"

"From my neck down I couldn't feel anything. To touch anything, I couldn't identify what it was."

Why were memories never numb?

"Did you tell anyone at Connaught Laboratories of your diagnosis of Multiple Sclerosis?"

"Yes."

"Who was it that you told?"

"John McCoy."

"Who was John McCoy?"

"He was the director of the Customer Service Department."

Jane looked at the jurors now when she talked. They were people like her—hadn't everyone in life suffered some injustice?

"Do you recall approximately when it was that you would have told him that?

"It was around '93, '94."

"Did you tell anyone else at Connaught Laboratories?"

"At that time?"

"Well, subsequently."

"Probably co-workers."

"Did you ever provide written documentation to Connaught Laboratories that you had Multiple Sclerosis?"

"Yes."

"Do you recall when that was?"

"It was after an incident that I had fallen."

"May I approach the witness, Your Honor?"

"You may," Judge Kane said.

"Would you look at Plaintiff's Exhibit 68, please. Could you tell us, do you recognize that document?"

"Yes, it's an e-mail."

"From who to whom?"

"From myself to Grace Cooper."

"What is the date of that e-mail?"

"6-8 of '95."

"Who was Grace Cooper in June of 1995?"

"She was the director of Customer Service."

"What was your purpose in sending this email to her?"

"It was in regard to the heat in the trailers that I was working in."

"What about the heat?"

"It was terrible. It was like being in a metal box with heat in it."

"And how did that affect you?"

"It was when I get overheated, it makes me not able to think straight. It makes me very tired."

"What were you requesting of Grace Cooper?"

"I was asking her to please get it fixed."

"Did she reply?"

"Yes."

"And what did she indicate in her reply?"

She read:

This week you came to me with your concern about the heat in the trailers. I hope this will be fixed shortly. However, I would appreciate you providing me with a written diagnosis of MS from your physician. Once provided, we can assure that your work environment meets your needs.

"And did you agree to provide that?"

"Yes."

"Would you look at Plaintiff's Exhibit No. 61, please. Could you tell us what that is, please."

"Yes, that's a note from my neurologist."

"And who was your neurologist?"

"Dr. Peter Barbour."

"What does the note say?"

"The note says: Jane Gagliardo is under my care for Multiple Sclerosis."

"What is the date of that note?"

"6-16 of '95."

"Did you provide that to Grace Cooper?"

"Yes."

"And as a result, was the heat in the trailer turned down?"

"It was actually the air-conditioning was broken, but the heat was working. It took awhile to get done."

"Would you also look please at Plaintiff's Exhibit 69. Could you tell us what that is?"

"That's an e-mail from me to Wayne Neveling."

"What is the date of that e-mail?"

"10-24 of '95."

"And what was the purpose of that mail—first of all, who was Wayne Neveling?"

"He was my manager."

"What was the purpose of that e-mail?"

"I guess I was giving him information on what I—the test I was going for."

"Would you read the first sentence of that e-mail, please."

"The doc seems to think that the problem with my eyes is from the MS."

"What is the date of that document?"

"10-25-94."

"And that was provided to Wayne Neveling?"

"Yes."

"Who was Brenda Berry, now Brenda Hanvey?"

"She was my supervisor."

"Do you recall during what period she was your supervisor?"

"Forgive me, maybe '94."

"Did you ever have discussions with her about your Multiple Sclerosis?"

"Yes."

"What did you recall telling her?"

"When I was applying to—for a job to go back to customer service and she interviewed me for the position, I told her I had Multiple Sclerosis."

"You told us about the heat in the trailer being adjusted. Were any other accommodations ever provided to you by Connaught Laboratories because of your Multiple Sclerosis?"

"Yes."

"What was that?"

"They had raised a desk for me."

"Okay. Would you please look at exhibit, Plaintiff's Exhibit 67. What is that?"

"It's an e-mail."

"From you?"

"Yes."

"And who is it addressed to?"

"Grace Cooper."

"What does it say?"

"It says: Thank you for looking into having my desk raised. It is much more comfortable for me. Thanks again."

"What is the date of the e-mail?"

"10-14 of '94."

"Why was it that you wanted to have your desk raised?"

"I was having trouble with my hands."

"In what way?"

"They were numb."

"Okay."

"I was having a lot of numbness."

"How often did you experience that?"

"Almost every day."

"How did raising the desk affect it?"

"Judy thought it would keep me from having my hands, you know, hit the top of the desk."

"Judy Stout?"

"Yes, she was a supervisor in the department."

"Okay, and she felt that raising the desk would do what?"

"Would relieve my hands, my numbness."

"How was it that she got involved in that in October of 1994?"

"Um, she had something to do with the company and the safety of the employees."

"Okay. Did she know the reason why you were having the numbness in your hands in 1994?"

"Um, she said it was carpel tunnel syndrome."

"Okay. Did you have any discussion with her at that time about Multiple Sclerosis?"

"No."

"Okay. Can you tell us in the time frame 1994 to 1996 what symptoms you experienced while you were working, if any?"

"Terrible muscle spasms, always fatigued, always tired, forgetfulness."

"Anything else?"

"And, of course, the numbness."

"Okay, Okay. The first thing you said was muscle spasms. Can you describe what you mean by that?"

"They're mostly in my back, very, very painful. It's very had to function when you have them."

"In what part of your back?"

"My upper and middle back." Jane studied the jurors' faces. For a second she thought she could see a few of their faces wince as she described the spasms.

"Maybe it's obvious to me, but can you explain what you mean by muscle spasms? What do you feel?"

"It's a mass of constant pain. It's just—it makes you unable to function normally."

"You said you experienced this during the time frame 1994 to 1996?"

"Oh, even today."

"How often would you experience that while you were at work?"

"Um, often."

"Well, that doesn't help us, how often?"

"Okay. They are always there. If you—if you want to touch them, you can touch them right now. They're there."

In their eyes it was if they understood what she meant . . . like a giant Charlie horse in one's leg or calf, the kind a pregnant woman might experience. Pain . . . wasn't it the one common denominator to the human experience?

"But in '94 through '96 when you were still working at Connaught, how often did you have them?"

"Every day."

"Okay. What did you do when you experienced the muscle spasms?"

"I tried stretching them out. I was going to physical therapy, and then I was told that stretching them out sometimes made them worse. I went to a chiropractor to get some relief from the pain."

"Was there anything that you did while you were at work to help you with the pain of the muscle spasms?"

"I used to lie on the floor."

"And where would you do that?"

"In my cubicle."

"Okay. You mentioned fatigue. What do you mean by fatigue?"

"Tired all the time."

"In the time frame 1994 through 1996 while you were working at Connaught, how often did you experience that?"

"All the time."

"Okay, and what did you do when you experienced the fatigue?"

"I tried to get as much rest as I could when I was home, but it just— I couldn't catch up."

"When you were at work when you experienced the fatigue, how did it affect you?"

"It affected me; it made me not be able to think straight. When you're very tired, you can't, you know, you can't—you can't focus. You can't think straight."

"And when you mentioned that you were tired and you had for-getfulness, were you referring to the fatigue also?

"Yes."

"And you mentioned the numbness. Now in the time frame 1994 through 1996 where did you have the numbness?"

"I experienced it mainly on my right side."

"Where on your right side?"

"In my hands, in my back, back of my legs." Jane felt the same numbness now as she spoke about those days, years ago. And for a sec-ond she wondered how it is that you know you are numb—there is something always inside that feels even when your skin and bones don't.

"And how did that affect you when you were working?"

"Well, it made it difficult to walk. The numbness in my hands, you can't feel what you're touching. It's difficult to type."

"You mentioned that you went to physical therapy. When would you go to physical therapy?"

"I tried to go early in the morning, or, you know, in the afternoon, but I always tried to make up my hours that I would miss work."

"Would you look at Plaintiff's Exhibit 70 please? What is that?"

"An e-mail."

"Is it from you?"

"No, it's from Grace Cooper."

"What is the date?"

"12-5 of '95."

"And what about your physical therapy was discussed in that e-mail?"

"It was in regard to the hours for my physical therapy."

"What about them?"

"They interfered with my work schedule."

"And what did you do as a result of that?"

"Um, I would either work later or come in earlier to work to make up the hours."

"Were you working eight hours a day at that time?"

"No."

"How many hours were you working?"

"Um, 10, around 10 hours."

"Even though you were going to physical therapy, were you able to work ten hours a day?

"Yes."

"You indicated that you first became employed at Connaught Laboratories I believe in March of 1987. Correct?"

"Yes."

"How long were you a customer service representative?"

"Until '88 or '89."

"Then what happened?"

"Connaught would get faxes from a company in Philadelphia, and they would send us this fax of orders that they had taken by calling like promoting the company, telemarketing the company, and I would enter that into the computer, those orders."

"Did there come a point in time when you also took a part-time job?"

"Yes."

"When was that?"

"Well, in the process of doing this I went to John McCoy, the director of customer service, and I said, you know, 'Are we paying this company to do this, to do this telemarketing?' And he said, 'Yes, I believe we have a contract with them.' I believe the name of the company was called Tel One in Philadelphia. And I said, 'Well, why don't we do it from here, you know, from in-house?' And he said he never really thought about that. So I said, 'Well, would you consider doing a pilot program on this?' And he said, 'Well, how would we do that?' And I said, 'Well, I would be willing to help with it, you know, to go work part time at another telemarketing room and bring back information how to set it up.' And that's what I did."

"How many hours a day were you working at Connaught when you did that?"

"Well, John McCoy went to his boss and they decided to allow me to work until 4:30 so that I could be at the other job by five. And I worked there until nine or ten o'clock at night."

"How long did you do that?"

"I did that for about two months, I believe, two or three months."

"How many hours a day were you working at Connaught?"

"I was working 8 to 4:30."

"After that two month period was up, what did you do?"

"I showed them how it would be cost effective for Connaught to do this on their own. And what they did was they arranged for me to do customer service in the morning and then telemarketing in the afternoon."

"How many people were in the telemarketing department when you first—well, let me ask it a different way. Was there a telemarketing department at that time?"

"No."

"Who else besides you was doing the telemarketing?"

"No one."

"And what did you do?"

"What we did was we took a certain area of the country and got the manager in that area, the territory manager in that area involved, and we did a pilot program to see how it—if it would be successful or not."

"Was it successful?

"Yes."

"And what happened?"

"It started to grow. We were able to promote people from the customer service department into that particular department, so that we would be calling outbound as well as there would be an inbound department and an outbound department. And what we would do with the biological product specialist (BPS) in that area we would have them give us a list of customers that they had trouble getting in to see, and we would call them on the phone and, you know, try to set up a rapport with them so that we could send the representative in there to get the orders."

"Did that ever become a full-time position for you?

"Yes."

"How long did you stay in that position?"

"A year-and-a-half, I believe."

"At the time that you left, how many employees were there working in that department?"

"At the time I left I think there were five or six."

"What did you do then when you left the telemarketing department?"

"I went back to customer service."

"By the way, I want to make clear, was that the name of the department? Was there a name for it?"

"For the telemarketing department?"

"I'm sorry, I can't remember."

"Then you went back into customer accounts, correct?"

"Yes."

"Do you recall approximately when that was?"

"It was probably the beginning of '95, maybe the middle. No, no, no, it was the summer of '95, I believe."

"Who was your first supervisor?"

"My first supervisor there was Brenda."

"She was the individual I think you testified that you had told that you had MS, correct?"

"Yes."

"Now, I'd like you to look at Plaintiff's Exhibit 7 please. . . . What is that?"

"A job description."

They went through the job description, line by line, and all the percentages dictated to each task she and the other CARs were to perform.

"And what percentage of time was assigned to special projects?"

"Five percent."

"Does the job description that you just went through accurately describe your job duties in 1995 and 1996?"

"Yes."

It felt like Pat's hands put her back together again as they waved and gestured.

The judge called a 15-minute break. Jane felt her lungs fill with air. She stepped down and shuffled back to the table. All she wanted to do was fling open the doors, barge into the hallway, and fall into John.

CHAPTER TWENTY-FOUR

Complications

—————✦—————

"Do you think that the truth really matters, Pat?"

"Yeah, I do. It might not seem so as the trial goes on, so prepare yourself."

"At first I was so nervous—I didn't expect that I would have to testify first, but I found telling my story empowering."

"Remember that, especially when Greco examines you. I just can't believe that he still doesn't get it—if a person with a disability can do their job with accommodations, they have to be made. I can't believe he is arguing something he doesn't even understand."

They swung open the doors and stepped into the hallway.

"How'd it go?" John asked.

"It was amazing, really. I really felt like the jurors understood me, that they heard me, you know what I mean?"

"One thing you do real well, Babe, is tell the truth. No one believes more passionately than you in standing up for what's right. Maybe it's because you had a lot of practice when you were young." He hugged her, swallowing her up with his imposing size.

They loitered in the hallway, watching a few jurors bunch together, stretch, walk, head toward the restrooms. A few turned toward her and smiled. Some kind of power, some kind of spirit guided her when she was little, protecting her mother, and it was the same now. As long as she didn't leave her mother's side back then, her dad wouldn't kill her mother. She'd tell the truth, and the truth always seemed to stop him—it shot out of her lips like bullets.

Truth . . . she remembered a few years back. It was Christmas day. She had to throw her father out of her house during the holiday dinner when he lost his temper and threw a tantrum and started to verbally abuse her sons. It always started with his mouth and ended with his fists. It was not the size of the man that counted, but the measure of his rage, she knew.

"Why didn't you tell me that your brother's marriage was ending? I had to hear about it from my sister?" His volume swelled with every syllable. Her mother shrank in her chair, as if she didn't exist in the room at all.

"He wants to tell you to your face, that's why, and he's on his way to tell you," she yelled back.

"I'm going to slap your face if you don't stop yelling at me," he said.

She sent her boys to their rooms, not sure what was going to transpire between the meat and potatoes.

"If you touch me I'll have you thrown into jail and the key thrown away, do you get it? You're nothing but a bully who is so weak that all he can do is hit women. I've had a stomach ache every holiday growing up, just wondering when you were going to start bashing Mom, you sick bastard. My kids are not going to suffer the way we did, do you understand?" She marched him into the living room, being careful not to touch him and opened the front door. "Leave."

She slammed the door behind him. The house rattled as if a minor earthquake had hit.

"I really thought he was going to hit you," John said. "I'd have to kill him for that."

Her mother stayed behind. John drove her home after dinner. They found her dad sleeping off a drunken stupor. The next day he called to apologize.

Standing one's ground is one of the scariest, most necessary things anyone can do, she thought.

Her MS is like her father, she thought at that moment, lurking, ready to blow at any time, without warning, like a tantrum of the body.

If only she could lead it to the door and tell it to leave and never come back.

Standing up to ignorance and bullies, risking your life to be heard, to win a decision that says you were right, or you were mistreated, and in the end, even if you won the battle, would all the people who were minimized due to a disability benefit? Or would it be only one voice, one victory, and in the end, be silenced by the abled?

Fifteen minutes clicked by. Jane followed Pat back into the courtroom, leaving John once again. Judge Kane called court into session.

"Mrs. Gagliardo, according to the Employee Handbook, there are performance appraisals every year. If you look at Exhibit No 57, it's your performance appraisal for 11-90 to May of '91. Who performed the appraisal?"

"Gerry LeBlanc."

"Who was he?"

"He was my manager when I was in the telemarketing."

"Would you look at Exhibit 56. What is that?"

"A performance appraisal by Brenda Berry."

"She was your supervisor in the customer account management department from the period of May '91 to May '92, is that correct?"

"Yes."

"You previously testified that Brenda Berry was your supervisor when you moved back into the customer account department in 1995. Does this help to refresh your recollection?"

"Yes."

"When would you have moved back into the customer account department?"

"In '92."

"Each of your duties is evaluated, is that correct, as we learned about earlier in your job description?"

"Yes."

"Would you read what it says under performance factor assessment?"

"It reads, 'far exceeds expectations.'"

Pat asked permission to approach the witness. Granted, he asked Jane to read a section of the evaluation. She read:

At the beginning of the performance cycle, each factor should be weighted according to its relative importance to overall performance of the employee's position.

"From May of '91 to May of '92, what category of far exceeds requirements, commendable and improvement required, did you fall in?"

"I fell into commendable."

"Accordingly, there is a range of scores for commendable, 1.8 to 2.79. What was your score?"

"2.78."

"Let's turn next to Plaintiff's Exhibit 10, please. Is that your performance appraisal for the period of May '92 to May '93?"

"Yes."

"Again, did Brenda Berry perform that appraisal?"

"Yes, she did."

"And what are the handwritten notes that appear on performance factor assessment?"

"It says: Jane needs to pay more attention to detail. However, when error is identified, she always makes the effort to correct."

"What is your rating?"

"Meets expectations."

"What was your overall rating from May of 1992 to May of 1993?"

"2.66."

"That fell into which category?"

"Commendable."

"Did you receive a pay increase in 1993?"

"Yes."

Pat directed the jury's attention to Plaintiff's Exhibit 15, and then asked Jane, "What is a performance award?"

"It was something that you were judged on if your performance was good. It was an additional bonus."

"Did you receive one for 1993?"

"Yes."

"Let's look at Exhibit No. 11, please. Is this your performance appraisal for the period of May '93 to May' 94?"

"Yes."

"Was this also by Brenda Berry?"

"Yes."

"Under performance factor assessment, what was your overall rating?"

"Commendable."

"Did you receive a pay raise for '94?"

"Yes."

"Did you also receive a performance award?"

"Yes."

"From October '94 to October '95, what was your overall score that time period?"

Again, Jane answered, "Commendable."

"Did you receive a pay raise that year?"

"Yes."

"Was this the last performance appraisal that was done for you?"

"Yes."

Pat requested that Jane read the section under employee discipline:

The company addresses performance problems through formal performance appraisal programs, supported by continual review and feedback regarding meeting job standards. Such programs provide a basis for recognition, problem identification, training, counseling, et cetera.

"According to the Handbook, if there is a discipline problem, the first step is performance appraisal, and the second step is verbal counseling? Prior to February of 1996 did you ever undergo verbal counseling?"

"Not individually, no."

"The third step is a written caution, correct?"

"Yes."

"Prior to February of 1996 did you receive a written caution?"

"No."

"The fourth step is probation, correct?"

"Yes."

"Prior to February of 1996 were you ever placed on probation?"

"No."

"Did you ever become involved in the disciplinary process at Connaught Laboratories prior to 1996 except for performance appraisals?"

"No."

Pat asked that the court look at Plaintiff's Exhibit 16, a letter from Dave Williams, the Vice-President General Manager of Connaught Laboratories, dated June 1, 1997, addressed to Mr. Pagano. He asked Jane to read it:

> Regarding the service you received on your recent order. Connaught has always been very proud of the caliber of people working for us and Jane Gagliardo certainly is a fine representative.

Jane lowered her head and started to cry.

The court waited as Jane worked to compose herself. Judge Kane told her to take a minute. A hush came over the room.

She continued, "'We are very pleased that individuals like you take the time to write and tell us about our employees.'"

"You received a copy of that letter, correct?"

"Yes."

"Would you read Mr. Pagano's letter please."

Jane read the letter:

> To Connaught Laboratories Incorporated, Swiftwater, Pennsylvania, May 18, 1987. Good Day—I would like to take a moment and thank you for my vaccine request—a single 10 ml of inactivated polio. As they say, a company and its products are no better than the people behind them. And my request was handled 'first class' by a person named Jane. She was courteous, knowledgeable, friendly and articulate; my order was taken, assistance in shipping was obtained, and the product arrived when I was told. No hang-ups, no problems. Living in Southeast Alaska, where everything comes in by water or air, can sometimes be a headache as far as trying to get something in a timely manner. I felt as though I was dealing with someone next door. I again commend everyone responsible, especially Jane, for the attention given to my order. It was a $50 order that received a million dollars worth of service. Sincerely, Michael M. Pagano, RPh.

Pat asked the court to turn to Exhibit 16C, a letter from Diane Turner, who had been one of Jane's supervisors. It was addressed to all the staff, dated May 18, 1990.

"Can you read to us what it says?"

Jane bowed her head and started to read:

I'm pleased to announce, that as of Monday, May 21, 1990, Jane Gagliardo will be assuming the position of senior in-house tele-marketing representative. Jane has worked long and hard for this promotion, and has proven herself to be not only upbeat, enthusiastic and easy to work with, but also an excellent telemarketing sales representative. I hope you will all join me in congratulating her and wishing her luck in her new endeavor. Congratulations Jane! Thank you, Diane.

Pat turned the page to another letter from Diane Turner to John McCoy, the director of the telemarketing department Jane had started, dated July 23, 1990. He asked Jane to read it.

I would like to commend Jane Gagliardo for her recent triumph. Jane worked very diligently to obtain an order of 7800 vials of Tetanus products from Bergen Brunswig Corporation. Talk about team work. Jane contracted Brenda Berry to make sure the management exception would go through, and that they would not be on hold for any reason. Then she gathered her facts; dollars, quantities, et cetera and approached Nancy Berger. After much deliberation, Nancy gave Jane the go ahead! Wow, what an order—approximately $56,000! I'm very proud to supervise such a self-motivated individual. Many thanks to Brenda and Nancy for their cooperation and team work. Once again, Jane has proven herself to be an expert sales support representative, she remains an inspiration to us all. Great job, Jane! Diane.

Pat asked to turn then to P 16 E, a letter to me from Angela Svenson, from Ocean Mental Health Services, Inc., Manahawkin, New Jersey, dated February 27, 1993.

"What does the letter say?"

Dear Jane, Thank you very much for the Connaught Labs gauges for measuring site of Mantoux tests. I do appreciate your generosity in this matter. I have shared them with the right individuals. Sincerely, Angela.

"Turn to P 16F please, an e-mail from Dave Williams to Jane. Could you tell us what it says?"

Dave, You received a call this afternoon from 'Jack in St. Louis.' He wanted you to know that Jane in customer service is 'truly an asset to the company' and 'certainly promotes good will' for our company. He didn't know her last name and didn't want to leave his last name. He said you wouldn't know who he is, but he wanted to compliment you regarding an excellent customer service rep. And then it says: Jane, great work. This is what businesses are built on.' No surprise to me! Thanks Jim.

"Who is Jim Brown?"
"The VP of sales department."
Turning to Exhibit 16H, Jane read another letter from Brenda Berry, dated February 16, 1995.

Jane Gagliardo. Great team work. Jane's suggestion to Helen Becker to contact a customer who was ordering DPT and who was not familiar with ActHIB/DPT resulted in the customer ordering ActHIB/DPT, Tripedia, and signing on to a new BOP. Brenda Berry.

"Could you tell us what P16I is?"
"It's a letter to me."
"March 10, 1995?"
"Yes."
"And who was it from?"
"It's from Bob Silverman, Vice-President of Marketing; Eileen Provost, Group Project Manager; Kelly Gray, Product Manager and Jeff Hackman, Product Manager.
"What does it say?"

Dear Jane, We would like to take this opportunity to personally thank you for your extraordinary efforts during the past week. We recognize that without your dedication and commitment, we would not have been able to respond as quickly and efficiently as we did, to the voluntary withdrawal of Phosphate Buffered Saline and IMOGAM. It is in times of crisis that we learn how important team work is. The Connaught team, with your help, rose to the occasion. Your participation on this team was integral to its success. Again, a big thanks to you, from all of us!

"P 16J, could you tell us what that is?"
"It's a letter from Dave Williams, dated January 17, 1996."
"Could you read what that says please?"

Dear Jane, After the hustle-bustle of the holidays, coupled with the difficulties associated with the weather we have been having, I decided the attached letter would signal the "official" beginning of the new year. I never doubted that we have the most courteous and professional employees around, but it is an extra treat when our customers recognize it enough to take the time to write. It certainly sounds like you went "beyond the call" and I wanted to send you my personal thanks. Keep up the good work! Best regards, Dave.

"At this point was Mr. Williams the President and Chief Operating Officer of Connaught?"
"Yes."
"Would you look at P 16 K. Is that the letter that he was referring to in his letter?"
"Yes."
The letter was from American Airlines Medical Department to the Chief Executive Officer of Connaught, dated January 4, 1996.
"Could you read the letter, please?"

Dear Sir: I would like to bring to your attention the exemplary performance of one Miss Jane Gagliardo of your staff. On two occasions over the holidays, at the time when it seemed most impossible to obtain large volumes of Hepatitis B Vaccine following the air disaster in Columbia, this lady's expeditious efforts provided me, in a very short order, with the vaccine I required. Perhaps as important as accomplishing the task was the manner in which this lady conducted her business. She's an excellent representative of your company who conveys through her friendly, pleasant manner the good intentions of your company to serve customers. Please extend my gratitude for your assistance during this time of crisis for my company and to this outstanding employee. Sincerely, Thomas E. Murphy, Area Medical Director, Miami.

"Do you recall what you did in regards to this particular letter?"

"It was a plane crash in Columbia, and they would not permit any of the workers to go up to rescue anyone without having this vaccine. It was Christmas morning. I believe the accident happened the night before. . . ."

"Would you turn to P 16L, please, and tell us what that is?"

"It's from Grace Cooper to everyone in the department dated, January 20, 1996."

"Would you read it, please?"

Congratulations Jane! Jane received a letter of commendation from our President, Dave Williams! Dr. Murphy, of the American Airlines Medical Department, wrote a letter addressed to the "Chief Executive Officer" commending Jane in her efforts over the Christmas holiday to supply him with Hepatitis B vaccine. Dave Williams copied in Merck so that they would know how well we handle their products. Great work, Jane!

"Turn please to 16M. Is that another letter to you from David Williams dated April 12 of 1996?"

"Yes."

"What does it say?"

Dear Jane: It is with great pleasure that I forward to you a copy of a letter that I received from Beverly Cudworth, Office Manager for Aurora Pediatric Associates. As you will see, she has some very flattering comments about you and the service you have provided—all comments which were earned by you through your dedication, expertise and hard work. We wouldn't be the company we are without employees like you.

Jane started to cry again but tried to suppress it—dammit, she was a good employee . . . she did her job . . . she loved her job . . . I want my job back.
"Take your time and let me know when you're ready."

"Thank you, and please be assured of my continued support and admiration. Best regards, Dave."

"Who was your supervisor when this letter was written to you by Mr. Williams?"
"Judy Stout."
"This about a month-and-a-half before you were fired?"
"Yes."
"Is P 16N the letter that was written by the office manager that is referred to by Mr. Williams in his letter?"
"Yes."
"It's rather lengthy, so I won't have you read it. Let's finally look at Exhibit P 160. Can you tell me what the You Make a Difference Program is?"
"It's a program where your peers submit your name to be entered into for recognition."
"Would you read what is says about the program in the Employee Handbook."

You Make a Difference! Recognized and honors employees of Connaught Laboratories, Inc. who demonstrate a strong personal commitment to the company's values. This is the highest award given to a CLI employee for excellence in one of the following categories: Teamwork, customer service, innovation, commitment to quality, community service and safety. Any regular, full time employee in good standing may be nominated for a Y.M.A.D. award by another employee, a manager or a subordinate.

"Let's look back at Exhibit P 160. Can you tell us what that is?"
"It's a nomination for *You Make a Difference*."
"For who?"
"For me."
"Who made that nomination?"
"Angie Zeglin."
"When was that nomination made?"
"May 3 of 1996."
"When were you fired?"
"May 26 of 1996."
"Could you read what it says?"

Describe why this individual should receive a You Make a Difference Award. Forward to Chris Kirby by 8-30 of '96. This woman has worked to keep two of my biggest customers happy. First, there was a billing discrepancy and my biggest account's Acthib shipment was not sent and without any notification and then had another shipment be withheld over this $1,500.00! This account will not—I'm sorry, this account will do about $250,000 worth of business and as you can see should not be refused a shipment for that small amount of money. Jane worked for over a month to try to get a 38-page audit of their account! The customer and CLI are working to see who needs to pay that $1500 and have made a difference to that customer with the service that we provide. Also, she has worked on a large credit for a mis-shipment that happened last year and wasn't applied properly. I think Jane deserves this award for not only excellent customer service but excellent teamwork in trying to provide me with information to keep these two accounts Connaught customers throughout these challenges.

"When did you learn that you had been nominated for the *You Make a Difference Award*?"
"After I was fired."

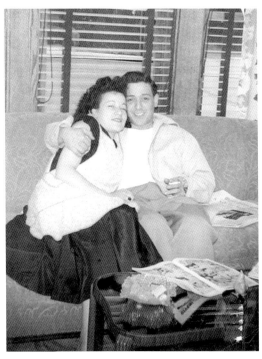

Betty Cervello and Chester Dovidio on the day of their engagement, 1950

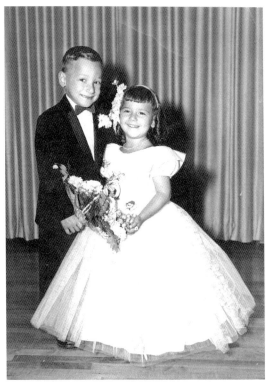

Dominic and Jane at Aunt's Wedding, 1956.

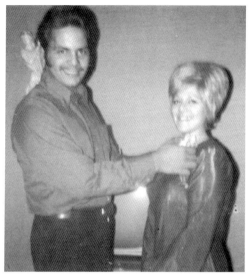

John and Jane at Jane's bridal shower

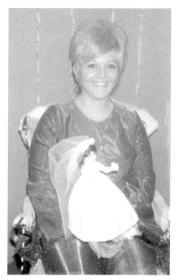

Jane's bridal shower, 1971

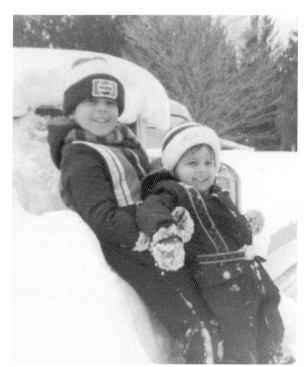

Joe and Johnny
after a snow storm,
1980

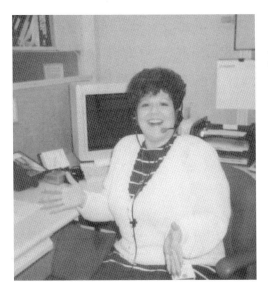

Jane in her cubical at Connaught Labs

Betty and Chet, taken during Betty's fight against breast cancer

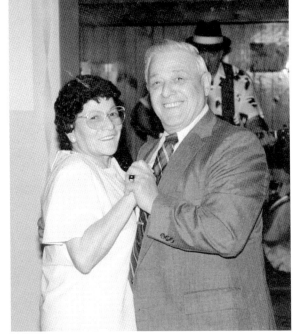

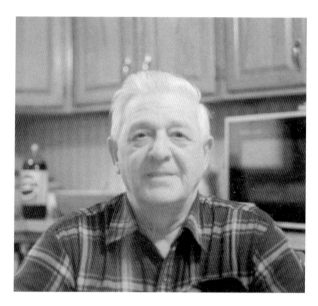

Jane's father, Chet,
March 1990

John and Anthony at a Fairleigh Dickinson University game.

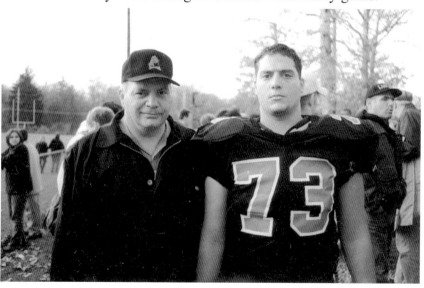

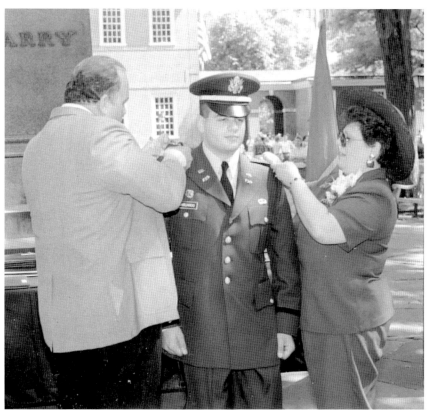

John, Johnny and Jane at Johnny's college commissioning

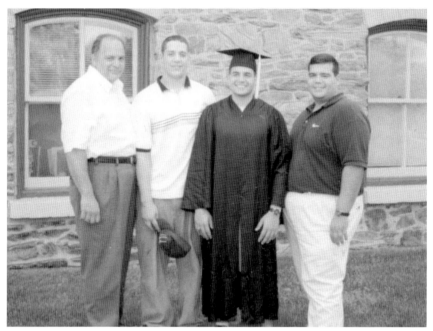

John, Anthony, Johnny and Joe at Johnny's college graduation

Jane, Joe and John at Joe's wedding

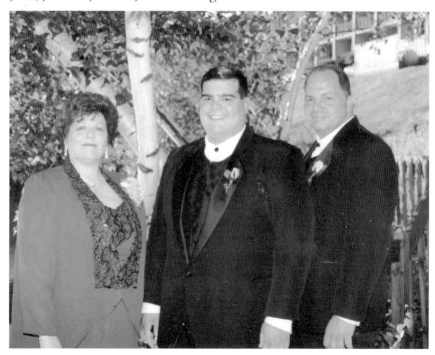

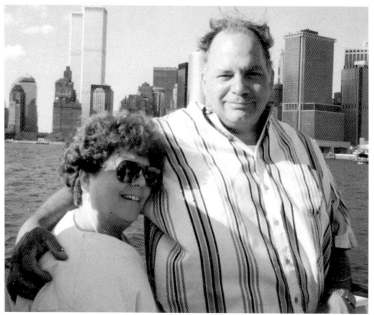

Jane and John on the Circle Line during the week before Joe and Mel's wedding

Jane and the attorney, Patrick Reilly

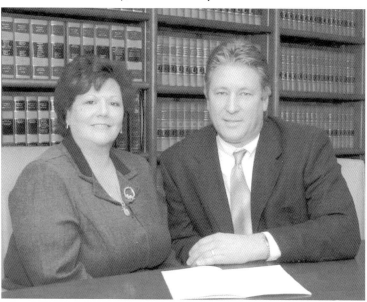

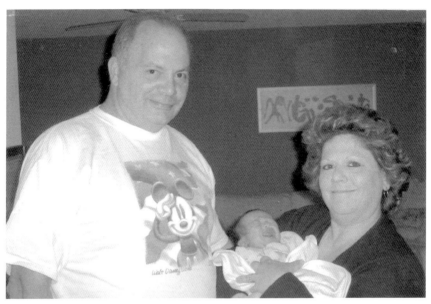

John and Jane holding their first grandon, John, August 2004

CHAPTER TWENTY-FIVE

Making the Case

The trial resumed after lunch. Patrick questioned Jane about the military orders and the difficulty she had had in fulfilling the orders on top of her expected inbound and outbound calls per day. Then he asked her about Judy Stout.

"When did Miss Stout become your supervisor?"

"In January of '96," Jane answered.

"Had you known Miss Stout prior to the time that she became your supervisor?"

"Yes, our children played sports together."

"How is it that she became your supervisor in January of 1996?"

"There was an opening because the supervisor left after having a breakdown of some sort."

Patrick glanced at the jury, an intentional pause, as if to signal the jurors to pay attention to the fact that an employee suffered a breakdown. Chris Kirby, sitting in the wheelchair to his right, was always in full view, a visual attempt to prove that the company was fair and didn't discriminate against those with disabilities, a sad, exploited spectacle.

"How did Miss Stout treat you?"

The story unfolded. Jane told the jury how Judy had singled her out and confronted her time after time, criticizing her work. Her work wasn't up to standards, she wasn't taking enough phone calls, how Judy nitpicked.

"Was she doing that to anyone else?"

"Not that I could see, no."

"What did you say to her when she did this?"

"I asked if there was a problem, and she said no. She just said that it was her responsibility to make sure that I was doing what the company asked."

"Did you ever have a conversation with Miss Stout about the fact that you had Multiple Sclerosis?"

"Yes, about two weeks after she became my supervisor. She asked me if I could get her information on MS."

"What did you say?"

"I told her I would call the Multiple Sclerosis Society that I belonged to, which is in Lehigh Valley, and I would have information sent to her."

"Did you do that?"

"Yes."

"Did you ever have any subsequent conversations with her about Multiple Sclerosis?"

"She made a comment to me that it made her uncomfortable that I had Multiple Sclerosis."

"When did she make that comment?"

"When we were alone in her office when she gave me tapes."

Patrick asked to approach Jane, and when granted, presented a handful of audio and video tapes for Jane to see. "When did she give those tapes to you?"

"During a verbal warning. She told me they were memory tapes and they would help me with my MS."

"She mentioned the Multiple Sclerosis?"

"Yes, she did."

"What happened to those tapes?"

"I gave them back to her after I listened to them."

"Did you discuss them with her?"

"Yes. I told her I didn't know if I had the time to listen to them. She told me to listen to them in my car. After I listened to them I asked her if she had ever listened to them since there were exercises you have to write. She said she had not listened to them."

"How did the discussion come up about the fact that you were having difficulty with memory because of the Multiple Sclerosis?"

"I told her that during one of our conversations, after a verbal caution."

"Had any other supervisor prior to Miss Stout ever questioned your memory or the relationship between difficulty remembering and MS?

"No."

Patrick then questioned Jane about the Biological Ordering Program, about what her responsibilities were as a CAR, and how there were periodic shipments made that she was responsible to ship out. Jane told the jury how she and the other CARs had received about an hour's worth of training performed during a staff meeting.

"You had a meeting with Miss Stout not long after this new program was implemented because you were making errors, is that correct?"

"Yes. She told me that I had made errors about an account that I was told to write up a history about that I had not been trained to know how to do."

"What did she tell you then?"

"She didn't care; she wanted it done."

"And then not long after this, she asked you to write up a standard operating procedure concerning the military orders so that others could be trained?"

"Yes."

"Did Miss Stout tell you during that meeting on February 27 that that meeting was the first step in the disciplinary process?"

"She told me that if I didn't start doing things right, that it could possibly lead to being written up."

Patrick pointed out different exhibits—emails and memos, including one from Judy indicating that the responsibility for entering military orders "will soon change hands within our department," dated March 8, 1996.

"From your meeting in February 27 until March 22, 1996, did Miss Stout bring any errors or mistakes to your attention?"

"Everyday. She complained that I wasn't stroking right. She would monitor me. She didn't like my tone of voice. One time she came to me and thought I hung up too soon from a customer, that I should have waited for the customer to hang up first and not hang up first, wait for the customer to hang up."

"Did you receive any training between February 27, 1996 and March 22, 1996?"

"No."

Patrick had Jane read the list of mistakes that Judy had listed against her from the February meeting and asked what Judy said at the end of the meeting.

"She told me that I had to make sure that I didn't make any more errors or it could result in probation."

"Did you receive any more training for the areas in which Miss Stout warned you were making too many mistakes?"

"No."

"According to the training schedule issued by Miss Stout, did any training actually happen?"

"No."

"From the time that you received the written caution on March 22 of 1996 until April 26 of 1996, did Miss Stout or any other supervisor tell you that your performance was poor?"

"Miss Stout did."

"What did she tell you?"

"She told me everyday as many times that she would see me in a day that I needed to improve whatever it was she was looking at that particular day."

"During that time frame did you tell her that you needed more training?"

"Yes."

"What did she say?"

"She was working on it."

"Let's go back now to Plaintiff's Exhibit 26, which you have identified as the notice of probation. What is the date of the signatures on the document?"

"May 1, 1996."

"Was anyone else present at this meeting with Miss Stout?"

"No."

"What was discussed?"

"That I made an error sending out the BOP and that I was making the Biologic Product Specialists look very bad in the eyes of the customer."

"Did you explain the circumstances of how it went out to Miss Stout?"

"Yes. I told her that the representative, the BPS, Brian, had called me with an urgency to get this product out and that he had had a very bad toothache and he couldn't go into detail but he was glad that I had it and to please get it set up and shipped, so that's what I did."

"What did she say?"

"She said that I should have looked at the date on the BOP."

"What does that mean?"

"What had happened on this particular BOP was this office only received orders on certain days, and by me sending it overnight to arrive to the customer, it arrived to them on a day that they don't receive orders."

"Did you subsequently learn whether they accepted the order?"

"They did accept the order."

"Was there any problem with the order?"

"No, sir, just that they were upset that they received it on the day that they don't receive orders."

"How did you feel after you received this notice of probation?"

"I was horrified. I had never been written up or put on probation or anything ever, and I didn't understand. I was asking her to help me get rid of the military collections so I could just do my regular job."

"What did you understand being placed on probation to mean?"

"That it was one foot out the door."

"How did that affect you?"

"It was very stressful. I had trouble sleeping. I couldn't concentrate, couldn't think straight. I didn't want to make another error because I liked what I did, I like the company. I didn't want to leave there."

"After you were given this letter of probation did Miss Stout come to you with any new concerns that she had about your performance?"

"Always."

"And in what way?"

"Anything. I wasn't stroking quick enough. I wasn't taking inbound calls fast enough. Anything that she could pick on she did."

"Did you see her having these same kinds of conversations with other CARs?"

"No."

"You were under the care of Dr. Barbour at this point in time, correct?"

"Yes."

"Did you ever have any conversations with Dr. Barbour about the stress that you were feeling?"

"I told him about the fatigue, and the spasms were worse."

"Did you ever discuss the problems, the disciplinary process, that you were going through at Connaught?"

"No."

"Why not?"

"Because I was ashamed of it." Jane bowed her head, caught her breath, to stop herself from crying.

"Did you feel it was justified?"

"No."

"Why?"

"Because of all those years I had given them, I just wanted a chance to have some of the workload taken off just so I could do my regular duty."

"When you say do your regular duty, what do you mean?"

"Just to be a CAR, just to take the inbound calls and enter the orders."

"Other than Miss Stout, did any other supervisor criticize you for your performance during this time period?"

"No."

"Now you know Miss Kirby. Correct?" Pat looked straight at her, as did Jane.

"Yes, sir."

"What was Miss Kirby's position at Connaught in 1996?"

"She was the person that took care of the human resources in our department."

"What did you understand that to be?"

"That if you had any issues or any problems, that she was the one that handled it."

"Did you know Miss Kirby during that time period?"

"Yes."

"Had she ever sat in on any of your meetings with Miss Stout?"

"Yes."

"Was she present at the meeting in which you received the oral warning of the written warning of probation?"

"No, it was a written warning."

"Miss Kirby has Multiple Sclerosis herself, correct?"

"Yes."

"Did the two of you ever talk about that?"

"Yes, during a private meeting."

"Before we get to that private meeting, at any time prior to that did you and Miss Kirby ever discuss Multiple Sclerosis?"

"In passing, if we were in the cafeteria, I would ask her how she was feeling. She would ask me the same."

"Did you ever discuss the symptoms that you were experiencing with Miss Kirby?"

"No."

"You started to tell me about a private meeting. How did this meeting take place?"

"I was sitting at my desk and the phone rang and it was Chris. She asked if she could have—"

"Your Honor, objection as to what Miss Kirby was saying, hearsay," Greco said.

"Sustained."

"Your Honor," Pat responded. "She's a representative of a company. This was a discussion that the two of them had about her employment."

The judge asked the counsel to approach. "What's she going to say?"

"She's going to say she asked her about Multiple Sclerosis and asked her if it affected her ability to do her job."

"I think he's right. Restate the question," Judge Kane said.

"First of all, before I get to that question, do you recall when this conversation took place?"

"It was after the probation."

"What was discussed?"

"She wanted to meet me in a private office."

"At Connaught?"

"Yes. When I walked in, I asked her if she had a tape recorder because I wanted to make sure I wasn't being taped. We both kind of chuckled about it. I sat down. She told me that she wanted me to know the severity of the errors that I was making, that they were very serious."

"What else was discussed?"

"We also talked about our MS."

"What was discussed about MS?"

"What it does to you as a person, how it affects your life. She asked me if I thought that the MS was affecting my job."

"What did you say?"

"I told her that yes, when you have been under scrutiny or put under a microscope with every little thing that you do wrong, it does affect you. She understood how being watched could be very difficult for a person to try to perform. Then I cried, and so did she." Jane could hold it back no longer. The tears came. She started to sob.

Patrick told her to take her time.

"She was very nice. She was very compassionate about the errors being costly to the company. We cried. Then the meeting was interrupted by a group that needed to have that particular room for a meeting."

"After the meeting, did she indicate what she was going to do about this?"

"No."

"Did she say that she was going to do anything?"

"No."

"Did she say she was going to discuss it with anyone?"

"No. It was a very emotional meeting. She didn't say anything like that."

"Did you have any further conversations with Miss Kirby about your MS after that time?"

"No."

"Can you identify what Exhibit 28 is?"

"It's an e-mail, dated on 5-21 of '96."

"That was eight days before you were fired?"

"Yes." Jane read the e-mail she had written to Judy asking when a coworker would be taking over the military collections.

"As of this point in time you're referring to the military collections, as opposed to military ordering. Had someone else taken over military ordering already?"

"Yes."

"You were no longer responsible for military ordering at that point?"

"I wasn't, but the two women who took it over really weren't sure on what they were doing, so they would call me to help them."

"Prior to May 21 of 1996, how much of the military ordering responsibility had been taken from you?"

"A couple of weeks maybe."

"Did you ever receive a response to this e-mail from Miss Stout?"

"No, sir."

"Turn to Plaintiff's Exhibit 29. What it that?"

"The termination letter."

"Prior to May 29, 1996 had you ever been terminated from any job?"

"No."

"How is it that this letter came to be presented to you?"

"I came in in the morning. Normally there are coworkers coming in. One person was there, and I said to her, 'Where is everyone?' She said, 'They have all been called to a meeting.' I said, 'What are you doing here?' She said, 'I'm on my way. I forgot something.' The phone rang. It was Judy. She said, 'I need you to come to my office immediately.' I said to her, 'Is there another error?' She said, 'Just come over to my office right away.' So I did."

"When you went to her office, was anyone else present?"

"Yes, Chris Kirby."

"What was discussed?"

"I went in and they closed the door. I sat down next to Chris, and Judy read the letter to me."

"What did you do?"

"I couldn't believe it. I said to her, 'Are you firing me?' She said, 'Yes.' She said, 'The error that you made was one that should not have been made because of the BOP and the DOC program. We're letting you go.'"

"What was the error that was made?"

"It was an order that I guess I had called, and they told me no product was needed and I had released it."

"This was under the BOP program?"

"Yes."

"Did you have any specific recollection about this particular order?"

"No."

"Forgive me if I have asked you this before, but had you received any training that was promised and planned on the BOP program and the DOC program?"

"No."

"Was anything else discussed during this May 29, 1996 meeting?"

"Yes. They wanted me to sign a letter of resignation. It was a five or seven page letter. I can't exactly recall how many pages. They told me that if I signed it, I would get $10,000."

"I'd like you to look at Plaintiff's Exhibit 65, please. Is that a copy of the document that was presented to you for your signature?"

"Yes."

"It's called a Release and Confidentiality Agreement. Did you have an opportunity to review this document when you were in Miss Stout's office?"

"No, I mean, I looked through it, but to read it word for word, no."

"Did you agree to sign it?"

"No. I felt that why would I resign from a job that I loved and get paid to sign something? It didn't make sense to me. You're firing me, yet you're going to give me $10,000 to sign a paper to resign? Chris told me that the reason that I should sign it is because this way when someone calls to get a reference on me for employment purposes, that they would be able to tell them I was a good employee."

"Did they tell you that this document contained a release?"

"No."

"Did they tell you that by signing this document you would be giving up your right to file a lawsuit against them?"

"No, they only told me that if I signed it, I would get $10,000."

"When you refused to sign it, what happened?"

"They got very angry."

"Who?"

"Judy did. Chris was frustrated. I didn't feel comfortable signing anything until my husband saw it. They were angry. Judy said to me, 'I can't believe you don't trust me, trust us.' I said, 'You just fired me. Now you want me to trust you and sign a document that I haven't even looked at?' Chris was sitting next to me in a chair and she put the pen in my hand and she said, 'If you would just sign it, it would just make it so much easier for everybody.' I said, 'No.' Then she made Judy leave the room so that we could discuss the COBRA, the life insurance policy, and such."

"Look at Plaintiff's Exhibit 3 please. Can you tell me what that is?"

"A policy procedure, corporate policy and procedure for termination."

"Would you turn to page three of that document, section V deals with severance and outplacement, correct? Would you read paragraph A, beginning with the word 'severance pay?'"

> Severance pay will be provided and outplacement services offered to all regular employees when the employee is involuntarily terminated due to lack of ability to perform the responsibilities of the position to supervisor's requirements. . . . A severance allowance equal to two weeks salary/wages will be paid to eligible terminees for each year of service with the minimum payment equal to two weeks salary/wages, and a maximum of 26 weeks. This is in addition to any payments made to regular employees in lieu of notice.

"Did you ever receive a severance allowance?"

"No."

"To your knowledge does this termination policy require you to sign a release in order to receive severance pay?"

"No."

"Turning back to Exhibit 65, page three, the confidentiality and release, does that document require you to give up your right to sue, for among other things, discharge from employment?"

"Yes."

"Prior to the time that you were terminated did you ever ask to be transferred to another position?"

"No."

"Do you recall at that time you were terminated what your rate of pay was?"

"14.60 an hour."

Patrick asked Jane questions about her current hourly wage, medical benefits, disability insurance, holidays, vacation time.

"Have you been able to replace the income that you were earning at Connaught Laboratories prior to the time that you were terminated?

"I'm close to it now, the income, not the benefits."

Patrick ran through income tax returns, showing loss of wages.

"Let's go back, Mrs. Gagliardo, to May 29 of 1996, the day that you were fired. Tell us how you felt."

"I couldn't believe I was fired from a job, especially that job. I enjoyed it. I loved the people I worked with. I enjoyed helping the customers. It was devastating."

"What did you do after you left Connaught that day?"

"Judy walked me to my cubicle. We left her office. I asked her, 'Is the security going to escort me?' because that was the normal procedure. She said, no; she said she wanted to at least give me some dignity. She walked me back to my cubicle and told me to collect my personal items, and there was nobody there. The whole place was empty. She said, 'I didn't want to embarrass you by having your coworkers here.' I said, 'I'm not embarrassed because I don't feel I did anything wrong.' She escorted me to my car. She took my parking tags. She told me to leave the compound, the campus. I left."

Pat looked at the juror who had been an insurance claims adjuster, who was visibly angry at what he was hearing, shaking his head.

Jane continued: "I pulled to the side of the road and I cried because now I had to tell my family, my parents, that I was fired. I had to face my kids. I was so ashamed of it. I was so ashamed. I went to my mom and dad's. I told them I was fired. I didn't know how I was going to pay for my kids to go to college because we had a plan that my pay was going to go—to pay for that tuition. It just took everything away. I planned on retiring from that place. Then I went home. I waited for my husband to come home, and I told him that I lost my job. He was upset. But it was horrible. It was horrible. It was horrible what they did. All I wanted was a chance, just a chance to do my regular job, that's all I wanted. They never gave it to me."

"Mrs. Gagliardo, has the termination by Connaught continued to affect you?"

"Yes, I'm very unsure of myself. I question my decisions all the time, particularly in the workforce. I constantly check and recheck so that I don't make any errors. It makes you feel that you're inadequate, that you can't do anything right. The day that I was let go, Chris told me I would never be hired there again because of my performance. I took a lot of pride in what I did. It affects me all the time. I'm afraid, afraid to make errors, which is a human thing. It took a sense of security away. That's what they did to me."

"Do you believe that you were fired because of the mistakes you were making?"

"No, I believe I was fired because I have Multiple Sclerosis.

"I have no other questions." It was as if their dialogue had been choreographed, as if they had reached a crescendo, a musical rest, and there was nothing more to hear.

CHAPTER TWENTY-SIX

Cross-Examination

Court resumed at three forty-five that afternoon. Mr. Greco started by asking Jane if she had ever read the Employee Handbook. He directed her to read out loud the disclaimer within and then preceded with such questions as to whether or not Jane had a written contract upon being hired at Connaught.

Jane admitted that she hadn't had a written contract; she had intended to stay with the company until she retired. When asked about the right of the company to terminate an employee, she answered that she had never considered that she would be fired since she had been a good employee.

"Termination never crossed my mind, sir, when I was employed there, until Judy Stout became my supervisor."

"Regarding your Multiple Sclerosis and your condition, I think your testimony was that your Multiple Sclerosis was suspected first when you were 30? Can you tell me a little bit about that? How did you come to suspect that you had MS?"

"I woke up one morning and I was completely, I don't want to use the word paralyzed, but impaired on my right side from my neck down."

"What did you do at that time?"

"I went to my family physician, and he referred me immediately to a neurologist."

"The neurologist diagnosed you with MS at the time?"

"Yes."

"Were you satisfied with his diagnosis?"

"No, sir."

"Why weren't you satisfied with it?"

"Being diagnosed with a disability or with a disease like Multiple Sclerosis, I certainly sought a second opinion. It's devastating to be told that you have a disease like that without being properly tested. I didn't feel I was properly tested."

"At that time, other than the one episode of your stiffness and paralysis, your inability to move about freely, had you had any other incidents?"

"There were things that would crop up, other incidents."

"Did you tell anyone at Connaught that you had been diagnosed with MS?"

"No, sir."

"Why not?"

"Because the other doctor that I had seen, as a matter of fact, I saw several, told me that if I had it, they felt it was in a dormant stage."

"Did you tell your employer at the time that you had MS?"

"I told them I was being tested for possible MS."

"Did the MS prevent you at that time from caring for yourself?"

"No."

"From driving a car?"

"No."

"Did you have any substantial limitations on your physical activities as a result of your MS after you were diagnosed?"

"Yes. I was out of work for three months. I had difficulty walking. I had difficulty feeling. You can't feel. When you touch things, you can't tell what they are. The best way I can describe it is, if I were to put my hand in my pocket and there were objects in there, I can't identify what they are. I don't know what they are unless I take them out and physically look at them."

"What did the other doctors that you consulted say?"

Pat leaned over Tullar, his co-counsel and whispered: "He's actually helping our case, inviting hearsay into trial."

"Dr. Friedman believed the MS was in remission, if I had it. I went to see another neurologist then when I couldn't feel my own skin when I dried myself after I bathed. I had no sensation in that part of my body at all, and I had some spasms in my leg. Then I went to Dr. Carrigan. He said I had MS."

"Were you satisfied with that diagnosis?"

"I knew there was something wrong, but I didn't particularly care for his tactics—the way he treated me. Before any testing he wanted to put me in the hospital and place me on IV steroids. I didn't want to be put on steroids. It has side effects; it can cause kidney and liver problems. I wanted alternative ways to treat it. I didn't want to take medications. He couldn't tell me that much about the disease. He couldn't tell me what, if any, alternatives existed. He just told me this was the protocol."

"This was 1985?"

"I don't recall."

"When did you start working at Connaught?"

"1987."

"Were you under any treatment by a neurologist at the time?"

"No. I chose an alternative route after interviewing others with MS. I sought chiropractic care. It helped the spasms, but I still had no feeling on my side—it would come and go."

"Were you able to work at the jobs you held before you were employed at Connaught?"

"Yes."

"Did you have any accommodation because of your MS at any of these jobs? Did the disease prevent you from doing your work prior to the time you got to Connaught?"

"No, sir."

Again Pat murmured to Tullar, "He doesn't understand. We never said it prevented her from doing her job, only that she needed an accommodation, as the ADA requires. This is unbelievable. He'll win our case for us."

"Did you tell anyone at Connaught that you had MS when you were hired?"

"No."

"Why not?"

"Because at that time the last doctor said it was dormant."

"When did you tell anyone at Connaught that you had MS?"

"I told John McCoy when I was working in the telesales department because I was experiencing some problems. Numbness, fatigue, were setting in. I later told another one of my supervisors."

"When was that?"

"Around 1994."

Greco went on to discuss the accommodation that Connaught had made—repairing the heat/air conditioner unit in the trailer. He asked her about the request for written documentation of her MS diagnosis so that the work environment could then be adjusted.

"Now, which neurologist did you call about that request?"

"Dr. Barbour, who was treating me."

"I'm going to direct your attention, if I may, to Exhibit No. 61. Now this exhibit looks like some type of prescription pad from Dr. Barbour, doesn't it?"

"Yes."

"Did Dr. Barbour send anything directly to Connaught?"

"No, to me."

"Dr. Barbour gave you this, and I'd like you to read, if you would, because it's short, as to what he wrote on that notepad about the information."

"He put, 'Jane Gagliardo is under my care for Multiple Sclerosis.'"

"Is there anything else."

"His signature. I guess it's his signature; I don't know.'

"I presume that's Dr. Barbour's signature as well. Now does that information contain any restrictions on your work as a result of your MS?"

"No."

"I think you testified as far as you know, Dr. Barbour never sent any information regarding restrictions to Connaught because of your MS, did he?"

"Not that I am aware of."

"Did anyone in management or a supervisory role at Connaught tell you that they needed more information about your Multiple Sclerosis at that time?"

"No, sir."

"How was your MS affecting you, other than the heat issue? You said your condition became exacerbated with increased heat? Is that correct?"

"Yes."

"Other than that, did your MS prevent you from doing your job?"

"No, sir."

It was late in the afternoon. Judge Kane halted the trial until the next day.

When the trial resumed the following day, Greco questioned Jane about her handicap parking sticker, her request to have her desk raised, about her missing hours at work for physical therapy for rehabilitation after injuries sustained in a car accident. He reviewed her work performance appraisals and emphasized where the management mentioned her proclivity for mistakes. Then he asked her about the military orders. He leaned forward, his eyes slitted.

"Did you ever tell Judy or ask Judy why, as you say today, you didn't get any training that you asked for?"

Pat studied the jurors. They appeared bored and restless; they fidgeted in their seats. Greco's attempts to discredit Jane wasn't working.

"No, I never pursued it with her."

"Weren't you concerned about it?"

"Absolutely   but I was afraid, Mr. Greco. Do you understand that? I was afraid to lose my job."

"That's why I have asked, Mrs. Gagliardo, if in the face of your fear, you asked Judy about the training?"

"No, I did not."

"In fact she says later on in one of the memos, 'In turn I hope you'll come to me immediately with any issues or suggestions that can improve your performance.' Correct?"

"Yes."

"Did you make any suggestions that could improve your performance to her?"

"Only in regard to the military orders. I asked her when was she going to take it away, so that I could just perform my regular duties."

"Because in March, more than ever, you wanted her to take that military away from you?"

"Yes."

"After the retraining that occurred on April 12, any additional error situations to occur in April, May and June would result in the company's move to the next step of the disciplinary process which is formal probation. Is that correct?"

"Yes, sir."

"Now I think you testified on direct examination that although that document is dated April 26, 1996, it was signed on June 1. Is that correct, Mrs. Gagliardo?"

"Yes."

"So you received that on April 26, and can you recall who was present when you received that?"

"Yes, sir."

"Who was present when you received that?"

"Judy and myself."

"Where did Judy deliver that to you?"

"In her office."

"It starts out by saying this notice of probation is with regard to the quality of your performance, is that correct?"

"Yes."

"Then in the first paragraph it refers to the written caution that you were given on March 22. That document contains a reference to an error regarding Brian Brogan and Carol Bryant [sale representatives], is that correct?"

"Yes, sir."

"In essence, do you agree with me that what they were saying was two things: The error was you shipped the customer's order to the wrong address, and you shipped it on a day that was not a receiving day for the customer?"

"Yes, sir."

"But it was your testimony on your direct examination that you felt that Mr. Brogan was actually putting pressure on you to get the order out. Is that correct?"

"Yes, sir, he had a very bad toothache, and he was in pain."

"Was it uncommon to get orders from the field or calls from the field and statements like they needed things right away?"

"It wasn't the normal practice."

"When it happened, though, was there a procedure available whereby you could expedite an order?"

"Yes."

"Would that expedited process allow you to fill orders on short notice?"

"Yes."

"Did you apply the expediting process in this case?"

"Yes, I did."

"But it went to the wrong address on a day that they were not accepting shipments?"

"That's correct."

"This letter ends by saying that you're on four weeks probation, and it has bad news in there, doesn't it, Mrs. Gagliardo?"

"Yes."

"Did the fact that you were going to be terminated or could be terminated cross your mind at that time?"

"Yes."

"Did Judy tell you in this letter that you're being terminated because you have MS?"

"No."

"In fact doesn't she say in the letter that you could be terminated and doesn't place a reason on it except for your performance?"

"Because of errors, yes."

"You ended up being terminated on May 29, 1996, is that correct?"

"Yes."

"Who was present at the time that you were terminated?"

"Judy and Chris Kirby and myself."

"Where did that meeting take place?"

"In Judy's office in another trailer."

"The letter that was sent to you, see P 29, Mrs. Gagliardo, if you would refer to that."

"Yes."

"That letter refers to an error in the second paragraph regarding biological product specialist Len Kendrigan, correct?"

"Yes."

"Did you dispute that error having been made by you?"

"No, sir."

Some of the jurors lifted their eyebrows, as if they appreciated that Jane didn't defend her mistakes, but took responsibility for them.

"Now does this letter say that you were being terminated in any way because of your MS?"

"No, sir."

"Did either Judy Stout or Chris Kirby tell you that you were being terminated because of your MS?"

"No, sir."

"Isn't it true, Mrs. Gagliardo, that you've never told anyone at Connaught that your Multiple Sclerosis prevented you from doing your job?"

Pat eyeballed Tullar and shook his head.

"That's true."

"Isn't it also true that the Multiple Sclerosis did not prevent you from doing your job?"

"My Multiple Sclerosis under pressure and intense scrutiny kept me from doing my regular job duties. It was very difficult to do that when you are constantly being watched and being told every moment of every day of what you are doing wrong, be it large or small. That kind of pressure, sir, and I hope you never experience having this kind of a disease, that you will ever go through anything like that."

"But, again, in the face of losing your job, you never told anyone at Connaught that it was the MS that prevented you from doing your job, did you?"

"Only during the private meeting that I had with Chris Kirby, and that was private between us."

"Now did you remember having had that meeting with Miss Kirby at the time you were being terminated?"

"It was before."

"It's your testimony that in that meeting you told Chris it was your MS?

"No, sir, she asked me. She asked me if I thought my MS was interfering in me doing my job."

"And did you tell her it was?"

"I told her, yes, I thought that it might be."

"Then on May 29 when all three of you were present and Judy gave you this letter outlining a mistake and carrying through on what she told you that if you made another error, you were going to be terminated, did it ever occur to you to say to Chris Kirby or to Judy, Chris, why I'm making the errors, it's my MS? Was anything like that said?"

Jane's voice sounded indignant: "I would never do that. I would never use this disease for that, never. What kind of example would I be to my children if I did that, if I used this disease?"

A few of the jurors nodded their head.

"So then is it your testimony, Mrs. Gagliardo, that you were not terminated in any way for reasons regarding your Multiple Sclerosis?"

"No, it's not true."

"That's not true?"

"I believe I was let go because Judy was uncomfortable with my having this disease. That's what I believe."

"Did you ever ask her that?"

"No, sir."

"Did she ever tell you that she was uncomfortable and going to terminate you because of your disease?"

"She told me she was uncomfortable with it, yes, but never told me she was going to terminate me."

"At that time of the termination you testified that you were asked to sign a release, is that correct?"

"Yes, sir."

"Refer to exhibit number P65, Mrs. Gagliardo. That's a document that was presented to you at the time of the conference you had with Judy and Chris regarding your termination, correct?"

"Yes, sir."

"You testified that you didn't bother to even read the document, is that correct?"

"No."

"I beg your pardon, Mrs. Gagliardo?"

"I skimmed through it."

"You had concern that by signing this document on that day, you would be waiving certain rights, is that correct?"

"Yes."

"Would you turn to page five of that exhibit. If you had read it, you would have noted what it states on page five. I'd like you to read that first paragraph."

Finally, Jane Gagliardo acknowledges that for a period of seven days following the execution of this document and release she may revoke the agreement and release the agreement and release shall not become effective or enforceable until the revocation period has expired.

"Now you further testified that Christine Kirby, who was at that meeting, took a pen and placed it in your hand and she told you to sign the document?"

"Yes, it would just make your lives much easier, everyone's life much easier. I said I'm not signing anything, not until I speak with my husband."

"Did Chris say anything more to you about that?"

"She wanted me to give her information so that she could tell people that would call about me, other employers. I don't quite recall exactly what that document was."

"But it's your testimony that Chris was trying to coerce you to sign that?"

"No one ever explained it to me. They just told me that if I signed it, I'd get $10,000."

"Then she wasn't trying to coerce you."

"Putting a pen in someone's hand? I know they wanted me to sign it. They were angry that I wasn't signing it. They couldn't understand why I wasn't going to. Judy's comment to me was, don't you trust us? They just fired me, and then you want me to sign a release?"

"Is that how you responded to Judy?"

"Yes, I did."

"What did she say?"

"She was very frustrated. I don't remember what she said."

"Now shortly after that you decided to take action against the company for what you believed was discriminatory action, correct?"

"Yes, sir."

"Your honor, may we approach the bench?"

Greco told the judge that Mrs. Gagliardo had filed a claim through the Pennsylvania Human Relations Act as well as ADA. The Pennsylvania Human Relations Commission dismissed her complaint without taking it to full action. "I'm going to ask her now whether she filed a humans relations claim and whether she knows if the Human Relations Commission made a finding they could not find under the Pennsylvania Human Relations Act."

"What is your purpose for asking that?"

"Your Honor, I didn't want counsel to offer these questions."

"Do you object to that, first of all, Mr. Reilly?"

"Yes."

"Why do you need to ask her that?"

"Your Honor, she's filed a claim under the Pennsylvania Human Relations claim and where that agency has already made a —"

"Absolutely not," Judge Kane said. "The only purpose I can think of you asking is to show this jury that some other right-minded person made a determination. This isn't involved in the claim. You can't do that."

Greco returned to the podium. "By the time you started your lawsuit against the company, Mrs. Gagliardo, had you already found employment?"

"Yes."

"I think it was your testimony that with respect to your wages, where you are now in terms of your wage compensation, is close to where you were at Connaught?"

"The day I was fired, yes, sir."

"I have no other questions right now, Your Honor. Thank you."

CHAPTER TWENTY-SEVEN

A Doctor in the House

Alan Tullar stepped to the lectern for the direct examination of Dr. Peter Barbour.

Dr. Barbour was small in stature, wore glasses, and appeared to be in his late forties. He walked to the witness stand with a quiet confidence, swore on the Bible and then when asked, stated his credentials.

"How long have you been in practice?" Tullar asked.

"I've been in practice of neurology for 22 years. I am an associate professor of clinical neurology affiliated with the Pennsylvania State University, Hershey Medical Center."

"At this time I would move to qualify Dr. Barbour as an expert in the area of neurology.

Judge Kane asked Greco if he had any objection.

"No objection, Your Honor."

"Dr. Barbour, in your practice as a neurologist have you had occasion to study the disease known as Multiple Sclerosis?"

"Multiple Sclerosis makes up a large portion of my practice."

"What exactly is Multiple Sclerosis?"

"Multiple Sclerosis is a disorder of the brain and spinal cord. It's unique in several ways. It's a disorder that is called a demyelinating disease in that the body identifies the covering of the nerves as foreign and attacks them and causes the demyelination as though you were stripping the insulation off a wire. A wire shorts out and the nerve system doesn't function the way it should. It's variable in what parts of the nervous system are affected. It's variable in terms of how it affects each individual. We don't know why people get it. We're not sure where it comes from. We have newer treatments for it, but none that are as effective as we'd like them to be.

"When you say none that are effective as you'd like them to be, could you expand on that answer a little bit?"

"I wish we had a cure, but we don't."

"What are some of the symptoms of Multiple Sclerosis?"

"The symptoms are very variable, and they are different in every individual. They can affect your vision, cause you to have blindness in one or both eyes. They can cause you to have double vision. They can affect your strength, your sensation, your coordination. They can render it impossible for you to walk or they can render it impossible for you to see."

"I think you have already answered this in part, but just for clarification, what is it about Multiple Sclerosis that causes these symptoms?"

"Multiple Sclerosis affects the covering of the nerves, the connection between the different neurons. So that if you think that you want to move your arm, there has to be a connection between where that thought originates and the muscle that makes the action occur. Within the nervous system there is an inner connection of these nerves, and if those connections are disrupted in some way, then the thought process never gets converted adequately to action."

"With respect to the symptoms, in your experience is fatigue a symptom that you encounter?"

"Fatigue is a symptom that virtually all patients develop and have. It seems to not matter how severe their illness is or what their neurologic burden is, how much or any plegia they have, how weak they are on one side or how numb they are. It's a symptom that's ubiquitous."

"Now with respect to fatigue, in your experience in treating patients with Multiple Sclerosis, does or can fatigue result in impaired concentration?"

"Yes. It's as though you were up all night and were sleep deprived and you're too tired to be able to focus on a particular task for a given length of time. Fatigue can interfere with your ability to do repetitive tasks. You can have fatiguable muscles or you can have sort of a general feeling of tiredness, which seems to be quite prevalent in patients with Multiple Sclerosis."

"Have you had occasion to treat the plaintiff in this case?"

"Yes, since 1992. I have seen Mrs. Gagliardo one to two times per year since then."

"Is there any medication which she can take?"

"There are medications that she could take. I don't believe she's being given any medications for her illness. When I first started treating her, the treatments were mostly symptomatic and were not called for at the times that I saw her. More recently we have discussed some of the newer treatments which have the suggestion of being potentially prophylactic, prevent progression of the disease. The science behind that is not as great as I'd like it to be. So we have discussed those issues, but we haven't embarked on any treatment as far as I know."

"What symptoms has Mrs. Gagliardo manifested over the course of her treatment with you?"

"She initially presented with abdominal pain related probably to spinal cord involvement. She had several years later an episode where she complained of some visual problems. She has had more recently complaints—"

Greco stood up and objected to Dr. Barbour's testimony of recent complaints. "The key date in this case would be May of 1996, and I would object to the relevance of the testimony of Dr. Barbour after sometime—after he first saw her, after the date of termination. I don't believe that any of that evidence is relevant."

"Mr. Tullar," Judge Kane said.

"With respect to that, Your Honor, the jury is entitled to hear exactly what kind of a disease Multiple Sclerosis is. It's a plaintiff's burden to show, first of all, that it's a disability and second, that she was regarded as having a disability. To that degree I think the jury is entitled to understand what the possible range of symptoms for Multiple Sclerosis is."

Judge Kane responded, "How does plaintiff's condition after the events complained of here, how is that relevant?"

"Fair enough, Your Honor. If you'd like, I'll confine my questions to the time period in question," Tullar acquiesced.

Greco, again with irritation in his voice, said, "Your Honor, may we approach the bench?" At the bench, Greco continued: "Your Honor,

I would think this would be difficult. Dr. Barbour didn't see Mrs. Gagliardo on the date when she was terminated. He saw her in November of 1996. I wouldn't have any problem with it if he talks about that record because he may want to show something from it, but my objection is—"

"I understand. Obviously this is a progressive disease," the judge agreed.

"Correct," Greco smirked.

"I'll confine my question—"

"To how she is presently," Tullar said, "and to the general question of her Multiple Sclerosis."

"How she was around the time frame," the judge further clarified.

"Specific to the time frame in question, that's fine." Tullar returned to the lectern. "Mr. Tullar, would you rephrase the question please so that the witness knows what he's answering."

"Yes, Your Honor. Dr. Barbour, during the period of 1995–1996, what symptoms was Mrs. Gagliardo manifesting or presenting with respect to her Multiple Sclerosis?"

"I have those notes with me. I saw Mrs. Gagliardo in October of 1995 and at that time she was complaining of variable vision in her right eye. I don't believe I found much in the way of objective evidence of problems, but that could be taken as a potential symptom of optic neuritis which is when Multiple Sclerosis affects the nerves to the back of the eye. She was having some muscle spasms of her right shoulder. Her symptoms seemed to increase as she became tired. Her hands and feet were tingling. Those were her symptoms primarily."

"With respect to Multiple Sclerosis, Dr. Barbour, is Multiple Sclerosis a progressive disease? Do its symptoms remain static?"

"It's an incredibly variable disease. I have had patients that have had one episode of involvement of their eye, blindness in one eye, when they were in their twenties and not have another episode until they were in their fifties or later. I have other patients that have had devastating illnesses where they have been paralyzed on one side and unable to control their urine function and get better from that and not have another episode for long periods of time. By the same token I have other patients who have developed one serious exacerbation after another and are neurologically devastated. There is a late form of the disease that can affect just the spinal cord and generally works as a relentless progressive disease. When you classify Multiple Sclerosis, you can define it as relapsing remitting, which means you have an episode and the episode gets better. Relapsing progressive in that you can have an episode that gets better but you develop neurologic deficit. And many patients later in their illness develop a relentless progressive form where they stop having the exacerbation and just get progressively worse."

"Is there any way to predict from one day to the next what particular symptoms a patient with Multiple Sclerosis will manifest?"

"No."

"Now prior to 1995 and 1996 when Mrs. Gagliardo first came to you, what symptoms was she experiencing with respect to her Multiple Sclerosis?"

"When she initially presented to me in 1992, it was a second opinion. She had presented elsewhere with symptoms that were thought to be perhaps Multiple Sclerosis. Nine years prior to that she had also had that diagnosis suggested, and I don't remember exactly where that was, but there had been a nine-year hiatus between that symptom and the symptoms I saw her with originally. The symptoms I saw her with originally, as I stated earlier, were primarily involving the spinal cord, and she had band-like pain around her abdomen or her stomach that felt like she was being constricted, which is a very typical symptom of spinal cord problems of this type. There were other symptoms that she had at that time."

"What about after 1992?"

"I next saw her in 1994. In 1994 she had come in again carrying the same diagnosis but had been involved in a motor vehicle accident. So the examination included things related to the motor vehicle accident which didn't produce much of any problem to her. As far as her Multiple Sclerosis goes, I thought her symptoms were quiet at that time, and I hadn't thought that she had had a recurrence from the episode before. Symptoms related to the previous episode had cleared."

"Now based on what you know about Multiple Sclerosis, during the time period that you treated Mrs. Gagliardo would it have been normal with respect to the disease itself for her to have been experiencing fatigue over this time period?"

"It's certainly possible. Fatigue doesn't seem to necessarily be a feature of how much Multiple Sclerosis you have. Quite clearly when you have an exacerbation, you tend to have more fatigue, and that can be an early sign of an exacerbation. I have patients that have very little in the way of deficit and continue to complain of fatigue. We have patients where fatigue in and of itself has been the basis of a disability claim."

"Do you rely on a patient to report symptoms to you?"

"Yes."

"The fact that your notes would reflect one symptom versus another wouldn't be dispositive about whether that particular patient was experiencing a symptom say that didn't appear in your notes."

"If what you're saying is if the patient doesn't tell me that they have a headache, I don't know that they have a headache unless I ask them specifically."

"Thank you for phrasing my question in a much easier way. Did anyone from Connaught Laboratories ever contact you with respect to Mrs. Gagliardo and her diagnosis of Multiple Sclerosis."

"I don't believe so."

"I believe you already testified to this, Dr. Barbour, but I'm not certain, so I'll ask the question again. With respect to fatigue, in your experience can fatigue result in impaired concentration?"

"Yes, I have to say yes to that."

"Would you expect that someone with impaired concentration might make mistakes?"

"Yes."

"No one from Connaught Laboratories ever contacted you to ask you whether or not Mrs. Gagliardo was experiencing particular symptoms or having particular problems with respect to her Multiple Sclerosis?"

"I don't believe so."

"Did anyone from Connaught Laboratories ever contact you and ask whether in your opinion a particular request for a modification of job duties was reasonable given her diagnosis of Multiple Sclerosis and her symptoms?"

"I wasn't contacted by anyone."

"No further questions."

"Thank you."

"Your Honor, may I approach the witness?" Greco asked.

"You may," the judge said.

Greco reminded Dr. Barbour of the deposition he had taken on August 25 and preceded to ask about how he came to diagnosis Jane with Multiple Sclerosis. "You testified that you don't know what causes MS. Is this correct?"

"Yes. There are theories, if you would like me to share them."

"No. When you are making a diagnosis of MS, does the name Multiple Sclerosis have anything to do with the appearance or the condition or test results of—that you might perform on a patient?"

"The name Multiple Sclerosis is descriptive. Sclerosis refers to the appearance of the nervous system when you look at it under gross conditions. If you were to cut the brain of somebody that had the disease, you would find areas of plaquing that are sclerotic and they would be multiple. Multiple also in Multiple Sclerosis refers to multiple within the nervous system and separation by time. So you have exacerbations and remissions that affect different parts of the nervous system at different times. You have one lesion at multiple times in different places. So you end up with multiple lesions with times."

"At the time that you first started to treat Mrs. Gagliardo did you take a history from her?"

"Yes, I did."

"At the time did she express to you in 1992 any cognitive disability she was having?"

"No."

"Would you refer to the binder I placed in front of you and turn to Tab 20. Do you recognize this document?"

"Yes."

"Is that your report of the July 8, 1992 visit by Mrs. Gagliardo?"

"Yes."

"Did you find Mrs. Gagliardo at that time symptom free and without any neurologic deficit?"

"I believe so. Neurologic examination is entirely intact is my impression."

"Did you in fact encourage Mrs. Gagliardo to do really nothing at that point?"

"At the time I saw her she was symptom free."

"In fact your report, Dr. Barbour, indicates that she had no visual symptoms. Is that correct?"

"I believe so."

"No loss of vision and that the patient feels fine."

"Right."

"No double vision, no paresis or other symptoms referable to cranial nerves, and you reported she denies fatigue."

"At that time she did."

"In 1992?"

"Correct."

"In 1992 did you prescribe any treatment for her because of her Multiple Sclerosis?"

"When I reviewed this note recently, I think in the beginning of it, one of the reasons she came to see me is because somebody had recommended treatment. Based on the finding of the MRI scan which showed some bright spots that would go along with Multiple Sclerosis, at this time my feeling was that to treat those white spots with a steroid was not appropriate, so I recommended against treatment because she was feeling well. I save that treatment for patients that are having an exacerbation in order to shorten the course of the exacerbation. It doesn't make them any better than they're going to get if you give them time. Without an exacerbation, I saw no reason to give that treatment."

"But clearly you didn't feel any of those types of treatments were indicated?"

"No, and there are some neurologists that might argue that those treatments are never indicated because they really don't change the course of the illness, although I'm not one of those."

"So if you thought that her symptoms were such that those treatments were indicated, you may have recommended them to Mrs. Gagliardo?"

"Yes." Dr. Barbour shifted in his seat and shoved his glasses up this nose.

"If you look at your notes, you see that you saw her again on April 26, 1994, and you wrote: 'Patient was last seen 7-92 for possible demyelinating disease.' So at that point in time in 1994 were you convinced that her disease could be called Multiple Sclerosis?"

"Let me answer it this way. One of the ways we used to discuss Multiple Sclerosis was in terms of possible, probable or definite. Possible Multiple Sclerosis was a young person who had an isolated event that looked like demyelinating disease, but you couldn't call it Multiple Sclerosis because there wasn't anything multiple about it. Probable if they had more than one event or you had evidence of abnormalities within the nervous system that were separated by space but without spinal fluid confirmation or some other more definite confirmation. Definite Multiple Sclerosis was somebody with lots of remitting disease who fit the tenets of Multiple Sclerosis, had laboratory data to support it. So whenever I see a young person who has had one episode, I am not going to call it Definite Multiple Sclerosis or even probable Multiple— well, I might call it Probable depending on what other associated things they had. So possible Multiple Sclerosis here means that my clinical suspicion is very strong that it is a demyelinating disease, but I don't have the confirmation of lesions that are separated by time and space."

"Your report continues on: 'Her symptoms resolved and no other symptoms have recurred to suggest dissemination of demyelination.' Is that correct?"

"She didn't have any clinical symptoms that led me to believe that she had more plaque within her nervous system that might have produced clinical symptoms. The feeling on that has changed as we have gotten to know more about this disease, and there is a body of evidence now that you can accumulate plaquing within the nervous system quite extensively without manifesting the disease clinically, and it's a basis for recommendations for treatment that have changed the way we handle this illness."

"Can you read what you wrote concerning the neurologic exam you performed at that time?"

"'Mental status: Patient was alert, oriented and appeared to be intact without aphasia or dysarthria.'"

"When you say appeared to be intact without aphasia or dysarthria, what do you mean by that?"

"I didn't do a detailed mental status exam that has some form like a mental state exam on her. Basically what I did in my examination of that time I would have talked to her the way I would talk to anybody and assess from my conversation that her memory seemed to be good, her behavior appropriate, and I didn't see any evidence of cognitive dysfunction at that time."

"In 1994?"

"Yes."

"Did she tell you at that point in time that she was having any difficulty doing her job?"

"I don't believe so."

"Did she express to you anything at all about her job?"

"I can honestly say I don't remember for sure."

"Is it fair to say, Dr. Barbour, that if Mrs. Gagliardo had said something like that, you would have reflected it in your notes?"

"I'm not sure I would have reflected it specifically as relates to her job."

"But if it was relating to her disease or her condition, it would have been there?"

"Yes, I might."

"In the last paragraph of that note on the April 24, 1994 visit you say: 'We would continue physical therapy,' correct?"

"Yes, for an injury as a result of a car accident."

"Did she tell you in 1994 that she was having any trouble remembering?"

"I don't have any documentation that she did."

"You say on your notes of October 23, 1995 that Mrs. Gagliardo was doing well until recently when she noted variable vision in her right eye."

"Correct."

"What were your impressions regarding that?"

"My concern was that she might be having a recurrence of her Multiple Sclerosis involving the optic nerve. That's the nerve that takes the light information to the back part of the brain where you process it."

"Other than the variable vision, were there any new symptoms of her MS?"

"I don't believe so. She had some subjective symptoms, including that her hands and feet tingled. She was complaining of some muscle spasms in her shoulder."

"The muscle spasms in the shoulder and the hands and feet tingling have been previously reported. It that correct?"

"Correct. I have 'not new' next to them. So I don't think there were any other new symptoms."

"And she noted no other visual change other than this sometimes when she was fatigued and in bright light?"

"That's correct. That's sufficient, by the way, for optic nerve dysfunction."

"Did she tell you that she was having any trouble doing her job because of vision problems?"

"I don't recall and I don't think so."

"Now as to the plaintiff's complaint of visual disturbance, you note in your report, didn't you doctor, that she was without much clinical evidence suggesting definite right optic neuritis?"

"That's correct."

"She made no mention of any trouble walking at that time, did she?"

"I don't think there is anything documented, no."

"Was there any mention of extreme fatigue?"

"I don't believe she reported extreme fatigue."

"Now your note indicates, doctor, that you had a long discussion with regard to the optic neuritis and the demyelinating disease, is that correct?"

"Correct."

"Did you ask her to consider going to an ophthalmologist before assuming that any vision problems were related to her MS?"

"Yes."

"Were you able to conclude, doctor, that those vision problems were related to her MS?"

"No."

"Do you even know if she ever went to an ophthalmologist?"

"I don't know."

"You scheduled a follow-up appointment for approximately one year?"

"Yes. In this particular case I probably suggested one year because I thought that the optic nerve problem was not going to progress, but what I tell my patients though is to keep me informed by phone so that they don't have to run down to the office every time something comes up, especially when I have established a relationship with a patient. It saves them time and money to just keep me informed. Had her optic nerve problems progressed in any way, she would call up and say, you know, 'My vision is worse, my eye hurts,' she would have seen the ophthalmologist at my direction. She would have gotten a visual evoke response study, which is indicated here what I was going to do if we needed to do it. But if the symptom cleared like many of her other symptoms cleared, I would observe her, and I think that would be appropriate."

"In October 1995 did Mrs. Gagliardo tell you that she was having trouble remembering?"

"I don't think so."

"At that time you observed her did you put any restrictions on her regarding her work?"

"I don't believe so."

"Was she able to hear as far as you know?"

"I believe so."

"Could she read?"

"I believe so."

"Could she walk?"

"Yes."

"Was she able to care for herself generally?"

"Yes."

"Did she complain to you of any cognitive dysfunction whatsoever?"

"I don't believe so at that time."

"Was she able to work?"

"As far as I know."

Pat turned to Tullar and whispered, "Thank you, Carl."

"Now you saw her then in November of 1996, but before November of 1996, doctor, and actually before October 23 of 1995, do you remember being asked by Mrs. Gagliardo to send a note to her employer regarding her condition?"

"I don't recall that."

"Your first impression in November of 1996 contained in your report, would you read that please, doctor?"

"'Probable demyelinating disease.'"

"Right, and you found at that time in 1996, in November, that her neurologic exam remained intact, correct?"

"Her neurologic exam remained intact."

"And the patient was without clear evidence of exacerbation."

"Correct."

"So at that time in 1996 then would you say that her Multiple Sclerosis was disabling?"

"No."

"Now your progress note indicates that since she was last seen, and that would have been October of 1995, that the patient has noted in the past weeks that her arms fatigue while folding laundry."

"Correct."

"Did she express any fatigue to you as a result of doing her work?"

"I don't believe so."

"Now your progress note indicates that: 'She feels her energy level is good.'"

"Yet she was complaining that when she did the work around the house, she was fatiguing."

"But she didn't complain to you that when she was doing work around Connaught Laboratory she was fatiguing, did she?"

"I don't remember discussing her specific job."

"She denies any new visual symptoms at that time, didn't she, doctor?"

"Right."

"She had no new numbness?"

"Correct."

"Now you also note that she had no other symptoms or problems."

"She describes a Lhermitte sign. Lhermitte was a French neurologist who described that when you have a problem with your cervical, your neck, spinal cord, and you bend your neck, you get a tingling sensation down your spine. It's a symptom that when a young person tells me they have it, they almost always have demyelinating disease. Even if I don't find anything else the matter with them, it generally indicates activity of the disease and what I think lends good evidence for why she was complaining of fatiguability with folding her laundry."

"Now in your earlier exam of October 23, 1995 she had noted at that time that she was having some visual problems. Do you recall that, doctor?"

"Correct."

"There is no mention in this note in November 1996 about those problems, is there?"

"Only with reference that she denied any new visual symptoms."

"Right, and she hadn't reported to you that her visual symptoms, whatever they were, had changed?"

"If they had been, it would have been noted. She would have been treated."

"Would you have considered her in 1996 to be substantially limited in life's major activities?"

"Only so much—"

"Objection," Tullar said.

"Your objection?" the judge asked.

"Counsel is calling for a legal conclusion, Your Honor. Dr. Barbour is a medical expert."

"Overruled."

"You may answer the question, Dr. Barbour."

"Do you want to define life's major activities?"

"Could she care for herself at that time?"

"I believe so."

"Was she able to perform manual tasks?"

"She could perform them, but she would feel fatigued, and it wasn't as easy as it had been when she was younger."

"Doctor, are most tasks or do some tasks become harder as people get older?"

"Not when they're 39 or 40."

"But your testimony is that she was able to perform manual tasks with some limitation."

"Yes."

"Could she walk?"

"I believe so."

"Could she see?"

"Yes."

"Could she speak?"

"Yes."

"Could she breathe?"

"Yes."

"Could she learn?"

"I would have to assume so. I didn't test that. I don't see why she couldn't."

"Could she work?"

"I would think it depends on the task that she was doing."

"Okay, but she wouldn't be unable to work at any task?"

"I think I would ask could she do the task as well as she should be able to do it."

Pat wrote down one word on a legal pad for both Jane and Tullar to see: *Beautiful.*

"Did she complain to you in 1996 that she was having difficulty at work?"

"I don't remember her complaining of that."

"So, doctor, in your opinion then as the medical professional, if we would define the major life activities as being able to care for herself, being able to perform manual tasks, walk, see, hear, speak, breathe, learn, work and think, if they are life's major activities—"

"Objection," Tullar said. "First of all, counsel is purporting to summarize a particular legal definition. I believe the definition he is offering is incorrect and certainly an incomplete question and therefore improper."

"The jury will be instructed on the correct legal definition of life's functions. Counsel may inquire of the witness as to the plaintiff's ability to perform these specific functions," the judge responded.

"Assuming hypothetically, doctor, that these activities, and I'll read them for you again, that the activities of caring for herself, performing manual tasks, walking, seeing, hearing, speaking, breathing, learning, working and thinking constitute for the purpose of this hypothetical question life's major—or major life activities, in your medical opinion was Mrs. Gagliardo on November 7, 1996 substantially limited in performing those activities?"

"I'd have to say yes if you define it as, yes, she could do all of those things. Could she do them four times in row?"

"I'm not asking about repetition. I'm only asking if she could do them."

"Objection, Your Honor. Define 'could do,'" Tullar demanded.

"The witness has answered. He has answered that, yes, she is substantially limited. Is there another question?"

"When you say she's substantially limited, Dr. Barbour, in 1996 did you note, or did you have any impression, that she was disabled?"

"No, because the neurologic exam appeared intact."

"Objection."

"Sustained."

"Did you conclude on November 7, 1996 in your office note that she was disabled?"

"Do not answer the question," the judge commanded. "That question was objected to, and the objection was sustained. Is there another question for the witness?"

"In 1996 did Mrs. Gagliardo tell you that she was unable to do her work at Connaught?"

"Not that I documented."

"Did she tell you in 1996 that anyone at Connaught Laboratories had told her that she was—because of her MS—she was going to be treated in a certain way?"

"No."

"In fact she discussed nothing about her job?"

"I believe she discussed nothing about her job."

"Doctor, are you being paid to testify here today?"

"Yes I am."

"How much are you being paid?"

"I believe $1750."

"I have nothing further at this time."

"Redirect, Mr. Tullar."

"Briefly, Your Honor."

"Dr. Barbour, with respect to your July 1992 notes concerning Mrs. Gagliardo's first visit with you, do your notes indicate anywhere in there that she was experiencing numbness?"

"On a regular basis for low back pain, cervical manipulation. She had some numbness of her right hand which was intermittent and unassociated with nocturnal acral paresthesia, which means that her hands would awaken her from sleep. That's a symptom of carpel tunnel syndrome, probably not related to the demyelinating disease. Though I have patients with demyelinating disease who have symptoms that look like carpel tunnel and aren't."

"Does the fact that Mrs. Gagliardo didn't have a particular symptom on the date of the visit mean that she wouldn't have those symptoms between dates of visits?"

"Oh, absolutely not. When I examine her on that day, it's just that day."

"Moving to April of 1994, Dr. Barbour. I believe you testified in response to Attorney Greco's questions that you did order an MRI."

"That's correct."

"Why would you have done that?"

"I wanted to see whether the symptoms that she was complaining about in the distribution of the eighth cervical root were related to a possible mechanical problem like a disk, as opposed to more demyelinative plaque in the area of the cervical cord."

"What were your conclusions?"

"My conclusions were that she did have some evidence of demyelination. She did not have a mechanical reason for it. But I didn't feel that in either case it was sufficient to warrant additional evaluations or treatment."

"Moving on to October of 1995. Dr. Barbour, the first paragraph in your office report you state that Mrs. Gagliardo becomes fatigued. Is that correct?"

"Not exactly."

"Would you explain that?"

"What I said was her symptoms seem to increase with fatigue, not that she becomes generally tired, if that's what you're referring to."

"By symptoms, you're referring to her Multiple Sclerosis symptoms?"

"Referring to all of her symptoms, including her Multiple Sclerosis symptoms."

"Which would increase with fatigue then?"

"Yes, that's not unusual."

"You have testified already that fatigue itself is a ubiquitous symptom of MS?"

"Yes, even between exacerbations, though worse with exacerbations."

"I believe you also testified that the neurological exam that you performed was intact?"

"Yes."

"Does that result mean that at that time Mrs. Gagliardo did not have MS?"

"Absolutely not. It meant that at that time I didn't see any manifestations of her MS. It's possible that the MS could be in remission or was just between exacerbations, but as we're learning from MRI scans now, patients continue to have activity of disease even when you don't see clinical manifestations of it."

"With respect to your October 1995 report, as of October 1994 when you saw Mrs. Gagliardo, was she exhibiting symptoms of Multiple Sclerosis?"

"I thought the visual symptoms were potentially due to Multiple Sclerosis."

"Did your treatment indicate any other cause for those visual problems?"

"No."

"With respect to fatigue, Dr. Barbour, in your experience as a neurologist can fatigue affect or impair the ability to remember?"

"Yes."

"With respect to Mrs. Gagliardo's reporting to you of symptoms again with respect to any particular office visit, does the fact that Mrs. Gagliardo did not report a symptom to you mean that she was not experiencing symptoms?"

"No, I'm completely relying on the patient to tell me what's bothering them when I ask them in an open-ended fashion what's bothering you."

"Would you consider the ability to concentrate or to focus a major life activity?"

"Yes."

Pat leaned toward Jane, and said, "This is huge, Jane, huge. He just established a new category of major life activities under the ADA. This is awesome."

"Finally, Dr. Barbour, with respect to the question concerning your fee, is that your standard fee for testifying?"

"No, not in court."

"Has it affected your testimony at all here today?"

"No."

"Is the testimony that you are giving today the truth with respect to your treatment and conclusions concerning Mrs. Gagliardo's Multiple Sclerosis?"

"Absolutely."

"No further questions."

"I have a few more, Your Honor," Greco said. "Dr. Barbour, referring to your letter of August 2, 2000 which you have addressed to Mr. Tullar. In the first paragraph you say,

In response to your letter of July 31, 2000 regarding Mrs. Gagliardo's Multiple Sclerosis as to whether it was capable of impairing her cognitive function in 1996, I offer the following.

Would you read the next paragraph?"

"My notes indicate that the patient has not had evident intellectual impairment from Multiple Sclerosis. My notes generally indicate the burden of quantifiable deficit has been minor. With regard to Multiple Sclerosis and intellectual decline, this has been shown to occur, usually after longstanding disease with significant exacerbations. The disease, however, is variable and may manifest itself differently from one individual to another."

"So regarding your impressions of Mrs. Gagliardo, you conclude, do you not, doctor, that she has no evident intellectual impairment from MS, correct?"

"Based on my examinations of her, which have not been in great detail, that's true. The intellectual impairment that occurs with MS can be very subtle. It might be more apparent to the patient than to the physician examining her and not something that I'm likely to pick up with crude bedside tests."

"Up until November 7 of 1996 had Mrs. Gagliardo suffered from any significant exacerbations?"

"She had two exacerbations at that point, visual and the band-like constricting pain. Possibly three if you include the episode that occurred nine years prior to '92."

"The next paragraph: 'Was the patient's MS capable of causing cognitive dysfunction and fatigue in the period of 1994 to 1996?' That was the question you were asked, correct?"

"Yes."

"Would you read the next sentence please."

"I guess it was capable/possible, but did not appear according to my records of that period. I believe that's correct in what I have testified here today."

"I have no further questions."

Tullar stood up as Greco sat down. "If I may, Your Honor. Dr. Barbour, with respect to your August 2, 2000 letter, the term cognitive function, does that embrace a spectrum, if you will, of symptoms ranging from minor to the serious?"

"Yes."

"In your opinion is there a difference between cognitive dysfunction and impaired concentration?"

"No, I would lump impaired concentration in the greater scope of 'cognitive dysfunction.'"

"Understood, but would impaired concentration be on one end of the spectrum and decreased IQ quotient, for example, be on the other far end of that spectrum?"

"Yes."

"Does the fact that your testing or clinical examination of Mrs. Gagliardo during the time period in question, the fact that it did not indicate evidence of clear cognitive dysfunction, mean that she wasn't experiencing problems with impaired concentration or memory?"

"No, I couldn't comment on her ability to concentrate based on the kinds of things I tested. I looked for much grosser kinds of dysfunction, and she exhibited no evidence in the brief period that I examined her that she was having trouble concentrating."

"Thank you, Dr. Barbour."

"Doctor, thank you. You may step down."

"Thank God there was a doctor in the house," Pat said.

CHAPTER TWENTY-EIGHT

Behind Enemy Lines

———✺———

Pat called Jane to the witness stand.

Jane rose from her chair. It seemed like a longer walk than ever before.

"Mrs. Gagliardo, let me ask you about MS. You have indicated in response to some of Mr. Greco's questions that you would never use your disease, I think were your words."

"Yes, sir."

"What do you mean by that?"

"I would never use it to gain anything. I would never use it to earn anything. I just wanted to work."

"Is your MS something that you discuss with people very easily?"

"No, sir."

"Now Mr. Greco asked you numerous times, and I think you responded affirmatively, that you've never told anyone that MS prevented you from doing your job at Connaught, and your answer was yes, correct?"

"Yes."

"Did MS affect your ability to do your job?"

"Yes, sir, it affects my life."

Patrick continued his questioning about the day-to-day expectations of her job, including the burden of the military orders, and further dissected the errors she had reportedly made, as well as her evaluations, and sick time she had taken for physical therapy.

"Mr. Greco asked you a series of questions concerning things that you could or couldn't do, including could you care for yourself, could you write, could you read and things of that nature. Are you able to concentrate?"

"Not when I am under a lot of stress."

"Are you able to focus?"

"No, sir."

"When do you have difficulty focusing?"

"When I'm put under a lot of stress."

"Are you able to remember? Do you have problems with memory?"

"Yes."

"When do you have those problems?"

"When I'm put under a lot of stress."

"Do you believe that if the military ordering and collections had been taken away from you, you would have been able to do your job? Do you believe you would have been able to do it without making mistakes?"

"Yes."

"Were you ever given an opportunity to do that?"

"No, sir." Jane stepped down as Patrick had no further questions.

Patrick then called Bruce Loch, a certified public accountant, to testify about lost wages.

Loch concluded that Jane's termination from Connaught was equal to an economic loss of $445,580 from the time of her termination to projected retirement in 2017.

After, Greco cross-examined, questioning Loch's numbers and conclusion.

Court resumed on September 21st. Patrick, John, Johnny, and Jane passed through security as they did every morning of the trial, emptying cell phones and briefcases and purse into the basket for the x-ray machine.

"I'm worried, Pat. What if the company retaliates against my co-workers who will testify today?"

"All I can tell you is that the judge instructed Greco strongly not to allow that to happen."

"Oh, so the company is going to listen? Give me a break."

"You are going to have to trust your coworkers to tell the truth, no matter what," Patrick said, retrieving his briefcase from the conveyor belt.

Guards nodded them forward. They rode the elevator to the second floor. The trial resumed.

Several of Jane's co-workers were called to witness in Jane's defense, each testifying that they had been aware of Jane's health issues, including her difficulty walking and fatigue. Greco cross-examined, asking each if they had observed Jane's blurred vision, numbness or tingling.

Tullar called Maria Durand to the witness stand, a registered nurse who worked as a CAR and a co-worker of Jane's. Durand told the jury she was aware that Gagliardo had health problems, including difficulty walking and fatigue.

Greco cross-examined, pointing out that Durand had not observed Gagliardo's blurred vision, numbness or tingling.

Other co-workers testified that they were unaware during Jane's employment of any complaints concerning her job performance; they knew that Jane had MS and had talked with her about her condition and symptoms.

Tullar then called Toni Fisher to the stand. Fisher testified that she had been Jane's supervisor when Jane became employed at a telemarketing company called Bil-Ray after Jane had lost her job at Connaught.

"Mrs. Fisher, during the time that you worked with Mrs. Gagliardo did she ever tell you how she personally felt about being terminated by Connaught Laboratories?"

"Yes, she did. She told me it was the most devastating experience of her life."

"Did you ever observe that Mrs. Gagliardo had performance problems with respect to her ability to make decisions?"

"Yes. I saw Jane as a very confident person. Yet, when it came time to make a decision, she questioned herself."

"Did Mrs. Gagliardo ever tell you why she felt it was difficult to make decisions?"

"Yes, she said she had never questioned herself before being fired. She very much sees her job as a part of herself. It's a very important part of herself and her life. She gives her all to any job."

Next, Tullar called Jane's son, Johnny, to the witness stand. Johnny had been sequestered by court order. He entered the courtroom wearing his Dress Green Army uniform, a dark green jacket and matching pants, highly shined jump boots, the pride of every paratrooper, pants tucked into them. On the left shoulder of his jacket, his Unit patch; on his shoulder boards, his Unit crest and rank, and one silver bar; on his label, a branch insignia, specifying that he was a Nuclear, Biological and Chemical Warfare Officer, along with his medals and his Pathfinder badge, and Airborne Wings. His Airborne Beret, maroon and worn folded down on the right side of his head, touched the top of the right ear, with a left eye flash. When the jurors watched him step into the witness seat, their shoulders straightened as if they were called to attention.

"Good Morning, Lieutenant Gagliardo."

"Good morning, sir."

"Are you related to the plaintiff Mrs. Gagliardo?"

"Yes, sir, she's my mother."

"Obviously, Lieutenant, you're in the military. What particular branch of the military?"

"I'm a nuclear, biological and chemical warfare officer First Lieutenant, Third Special Forces Group."

"How long have you been on active duty?"

"Approximately two years."

"Prior to active duty in the military what was your educational background?"

"I was a student at Widener University as well as an ROTC cadet."

"Did you obtain a degree from Widener?"

"Yes, in criminal justice."

"When did you graduate from Widener?"

"May of 1998."

"While you were attending Widener where did you reside?"

"At my parents' home, with my mom and dad."

"Did there ever come a time that you learned that your mom had Multiple Sclerosis?"

"Yes, sir."

"How did you learn that?"

"Mom sat the three of us down and pretty much broke the news to us all together."

"What was her emotional state when she told you she had MS?"

"I don't think she wanted us to see her upset at that point."

"What was your reaction when you heard?"

"I had no idea exactly what it was. I had assumed that since Mom had gathered the three of us together, my two brothers and myself, that it was more than likely something serious. I really didn't know what it was all about."

"Do you remember when this was?"

"I was in college at the time."

"During the time that you were going to school and living at home did you ever observe any problems that your mom was having that you thought were related to the MS?"

"Mom has always been a very outgoing, energetic person. I could tell that going to school when I came back from school after a few months, Mom was definitely beginning to slow down a little bit. She always got through it and she did everything, but it took her a lot more time, and she would get fatigued very easily."

"When you say it slowed her down, did you ever notice problems with her balance?"

"When we would be out or into the store, we'd be walking for a while, and I would notice that she would have to lean against something or she would hold my arm or the arm of my father or one of my brothers just for a couple of minutes. She said she needed a little rest. She would get tired and that sort of thing."

"With respect to the fatigue, what exactly did you notice? How did you notice that she was fatigued?"

"She would come in the living room, and she would say, 'I just have to sit down,' and sometimes she wouldn't get back up because she was tired. She would go right to bed if it was in the evening or we would go in and finish whatever Mom had started. You could tell there was something wrong, and there was definitely something affecting Mom."

"Did your mom ever talk to you about her job at Connaught Laboratories?"

"A little bit."

"What would she tell you?"

"With going in the military, Mom would tell me that the military had ordered a large quantity of vaccines, other than the basic run-of-the-mill stuff, nothing."

"Did she like her job?"

"Yes, she did."

"How do you know that?"

"She would tell us that she could feel that she was making a difference with someone. Specifically I can remember when Mom would deal with the rabies vaccines, and she would have a beeper and it would go off, on Saturday evening or Saturday afternoon, and Mom would be responsible for rushing this vaccine to Wyoming or Utah or wherever, and you could tell she was happy. She would say, 'I made a difference today and I got this vaccine to someone who really needed it.'"

"Did you ever notice any problems with your mom's concentration or with her ability to focus again during that time period when you were living at home?"

"It's hard to tell with Mom. She doesn't like to show anyone that she's having problems. My two brothers, myself and my father are extremely protective of my mother. So whenever something bothers her, we feel responsible to find out what it is and make sure that it doesn't bother her anymore. And with the MS it's difficult because there is nothing we can do about it. But you could tell there was something going on in Mom's mind, something that was bothering her, that she wasn't always able to focus on everything that she used to be able to."

"So even if she didn't talk to you or mention anything to you, did you yourself notice?"

"Yes, yes, sir."

"Those are problems—she would have problems focusing sometimes?"

"Yes, sir."

"Were you living at home when your mom was fired by Connaught Laboratories?"

"Yes, sir."

"How did you hear about your mom being fired?"

"She had told me that she was fired."

"What was she like emotionally when she told you that?"

"I believe initially Mom was shocked because she had enjoyed the job, and I truly believe she was a little embarrassed to tell us that she had been fired. She was definitely upset about it, absolutely."

"Did you notice any changes in your mom after she was fired?"

"It seemed that on top of the MS, Mom was stressed about the whole thing. I think it was a big pride issue with Mom. She has always been a hard worker, and she had never been fired from anything before."

"So when you say there was stressed, what exactly did you see in terms of your mom's emotional state?"

"She just wasn't as outgoing as she had been. Mom has always had the spring in her step, for lack of a better phrase, and it was something that was missing, something was definitely missing following her being fired from Connaught."

"Has that spring come back today?"

"No, no, sir."

"No further questions at this time."

Mr. Greco stood up and stepped to the lectern.

"Thank you, Your Honor. Good Morning, Lieutenant Gagliardo. Your mother is working now, isn't she?"

"Yes, sir."

"Is she happy with her job now?"

"I haven't spoken with Mom about her job in quite some time."

"She's your mother and you love her, don't you?"

"Yes, sir."

"And you'd do anything for her?"

"I would not do anything for her. I would not lie in a court of law for my mother or my father." From Johnny's face, it appeared as if he had just landed behind enemy lines.

Greco's jaw sagged; his eyes widened. He looked as if he had lost his way. "Short of lying, would you do anything for them?"

"Depending on the circumstances."

"You felt, I think your testimony was, that when you, your father and your brothers feel that something goes wrong with your mother, that you want to find out what it is. Is that your testimony?"

"Yes, sir."

"Did you ever call anyone at Connaught to find out anything about her termination?"

"No, sir."

"No further questions, Your Honor."

The judge called a recess. Johnny stepped down, thanked the judge and jury. He approached Jane and helped her up before hugging her. They walked down the aisle and into the hallway that now smelled of soup cooking somewhere in the building.

"I have got to tell you, Mom, when their lawyer was questioning me, the first thing I noticed was a blue *Bic* pen that was sitting on the front of the stand. It was uncapped and the point was exposed. I was curious as to why it was there. I looked at the jury. It looked as though up to three jurors were prior service. I saw their eyes, they knew what the jump boots, beret and overall attitude meant. When he asked, 'LT Gagliardo, do you love your mother?' I kept thinking that I could easily cover the twelve or so feet between my seat and the lectern in less than five seconds before any one would have an opportunity to stop me. On my way, I'd grab the pen, I would drive it into the lawyer's throat right above his adam's apple, nice and clean. I wanted him to have the worst day of his life for trying to hurt you, Mom. I hope he's updating his resume. He picked the wrong fight with the wrong family."

"Plaintiff calls John Gagliardo, Sr."

John entered the room, a huge physical presence.

Tullar established that John, age forty-seven, was Jane's husband, and that they had been married for thirty years.

"Mr. Gagliardo, there came a point in time when your wife was diagnosed with Multiple Sclerosis, correct?"

"Yes."

"Have you had an opportunity to observe the effect that the MS has had upon her?"

"Yes, I have."

"Can you describe the effects of the MS on your wife as you have observed them?"

"She has periods of fatigue. She does have forgetfulness, which usually happens when she's tired, and that's when she does have problem with memory, to some degree. It upsets her when she's in this state. She does have some shaking when she's fatigued."

"Is there anything that brings on the fatigue that you're aware of based on what you have observed?"

"Stress, any type of stress."

"You indicated that when she becomes fatigued, she has difficulty remembering, correct?"

"Yes."

"Does she have difficulty concentrating?"

"Yes."

"And focusing?"

"Yes."

"You have observed that?"

"Yes, sir."

"In addition to that has your wife ever discussed with you how the MS makes her feel?"

"I don't know if the proper word is ashamed, but possibly embarrassed by it. She doesn't really like to discuss it."

"Is it something that she discusses easily with others?"

"No."

"Is it something she volunteers to others?"

"Not really."

"Does she ever use it as an excuse for anything?"

"No."

"Does she ever tell you physically the effects that the MS have on her?"

"At times she'll tell me she's having back spasms, things of that nature, and I massage her back and make her feel a little better if I can."

"Describe for us what your wife was like prior to 1996."

"My wife was fairly involved with our kids being in sports. She enjoyed that. She enjoyed her job; she liked it very much. I felt she was over-dedicated. But in general I guess you could say we were happy, the both of us, with our life and our lifestyle."

"Did she ever discuss with you how she felt about work?"

"She loved her job."

"How do you know that?"

"Most people are a little apprehensive on a Monday morning. She was happy it was Monday morning to go to work because she liked her job."

The jurors laughed, as if they related to the dread of work.

"Was she proud of what she did?"

"Yes, she was."

"Did that change at any time?"

"Yes, in the beginning of 1996."

"What changed?"

"She had a new supervisor, and she felt that she was being scrutinized."

"Did she tell you how she was feeling as a result of what was going on at work?"

"She felt like more stress, more pressure, was on her."

"How was that affecting her?"

"Obviously she was a little more nervous, a little more tired, still enjoyed her job though, and I could just tell that she was under pressure. I have been with the woman thirty years; I know what she's like."

"Do the two of you have a close relationship?"

"Yes, sir."

"Do you discuss things amongst yourselves? Do you share feelings?"

"We certainly do."

"There came a point in time when she received an oral warning about mistakes she was making. Did you learn of that?"

"Yes, sir."

"How did you learn of that?"

"She came home and explained to me that she received an oral warning for something she had supposedly done wrong at work. She was very upset. She was not happy that she made an error. She felt it was a bad reflection on her job. She came home that day and talked about it. Her demeanor just changed. She was upset."

"Did you learn that she had received a written caution?"

"Yes. She told me about it. She told me she received a written caution, she really didn't understand it, why all of a sudden she was getting picked on. She said other people in her department were making mistakes and they weren't getting this type of treatment. She again felt Judy Stout was focusing on her."

"Did you notice how it affected her?"

"Yes, she seemed upset by it, and she seemed to put a lot of pressure on herself not to make any more errors."

"In your experience with your wife when she puts pressure on herself, how does that affect her?"

"Naturally, like most people they become a little short tempered. She then becomes more fatigued."

"Did you learn that she was placed on probation?"

"Yes, she came home and told me. She was really upset about it."

"When you say she was upset, how did you know she was upset?"

"I could tell when I walked in the door with just one look at my wife. I think most couples can tell what mood they are in, and I knew something was wrong. I could tell by the look on her face. She couldn't understand it, where this had come from because up until this point in regards to Judy, as her supervisor/manager, she had been receiving commendations from even the president of the company that she was an asset, and then all of a sudden to go in this direction just seemed like a complete about face."

"Did it affect her in any physical way that you were able to observe?"

"Sometimes she would get so upset that she would develop shaking, which I didn't want to bring up to her because she would be embarrassed by it."

"Finally, when did you learn that your wife had been fired by Connaught?"

"On the day of her firing. I asked her what happened, and she said Judy fired her, that they brought her into an office, and Chris Kirby was there. They wanted her to sign this document, waiver or something, and told her that if she signed it, in the way I read the document, 'If you keep your mouth shut, we'll pay you $10,000.'"

"Was she upset?"

"She was upset—she had rapid speech, anger, frustration, bewilderment. She was just totally taken aback by it. She felt that she did her job and to the best of her ability and was singled out and terminated."

"How long did that anger and frustration and bewilderment continue?"

"For a while. If I were to put a time frame on it, I don't think it's ever gone."

"In your opinion, is she still suffering from the effects of that?"

"Yes."

"In what way?"

"I believe my wife, prior to this termination, was a fairly directed person, knew where she wanted to go, was a decision maker. Now she's very tentative and seems to double check her decisions even in the household. She's very unsure of herself anymore."

"Emotionally is she still affected by it?"

"Yes, sir. She has moments where's she crying when she thinks about Connaught. Obviously with the events going on, this has been a pretty hard time for her. She's fatigued obviously the last couple of days especially. She I think down deep inside of her she's still in to some degree some type of shock about it."

"Why do you say that?"

"Because she feels she did nothing wrong and she was fired."

"Is she the same person she was prior to being fired?"

"In no way, shape or form."

"After she was terminated by Connaught did she look for other work?"

"Yes, but her heart wasn't in it. She was still pretty disillusioned I'd guess you could say. She started looking for another job within a week, but it took her a year to find a job."

"Was she emotionally ready to return to another job?"

"No. She wasn't herself. I don't know if I could describe it into words; she seemed off-centered, disillusioned, just shocked. I had never seen her like this before. The zing has gone from her step."

"Is working important to her?"

"Yes."

"All right, thank you."

The Court called Mr. Greco.

"I have no questions, Your Honor."

CHAPTER TWENTY-NINE

Enemy Territory

The court decided after some discussion among the lawyers and judge that Chris Kirby would testify from her wheelchair. Her nurse wheeled her to the front of the witness stand where she swore to tell the truth. Upon Patrick's questioning, Kirby explained that she was currently a website coordinator for the company.

"In 1995 and 1996 you were an employee relations manager, correct?" Patrick's voice was gentle. It was clear that Connaught was exploiting her and he wanted to be careful not to do the same.

"I was manager of employee communications and human resources information systems."

"You were responsible for the finance administration and information systems, and your area of responsibility covered customer account representatives, did it not?"

"Yes."

Patrick drew attention to the Employee Handbook, focusing on what her position entailed and the company's policies.

"The Equal Employment Opportunity policy would cover, among other things, the Americans with Disabilities Act?"

"At that time, yes."

"Do you know if the Americans with Disabilities Act was enacted in 1990?"

"I don't know that for a fact, but I believe so."

"Do you know after 1990, up to the time frame of 1996, whether or not the equal employment opportunity policy of Connaught Laboratories was amended to reflect inclusion of the Americans with Disabilities Act?"

"Again I don't know that for a fact, but I would expect that it would be. At some point we wrote a separate policy for ADA, and I don't know the date for that."

"The policy statement states:

Connaught Laboratories, Inc. is committed to providing equal employment opportunities for all our employees. Practices and decisions relating to all aspects of the company's relationship to its employees will always be conducted without regard to race, color, religion, sex, national origin, age, handicap or veteran status.

Is that what it says?"

"Yes."

"Did you agree with that in 1995 and 1996?"

"Yes."

"What training did you, as a member of the human resources department, receive on the Americans with Disabilities Act prior to 1996?"

"We, as I recall, we had regular staff meetings amongst the human resources professionals, and that would have been a topic covered at our staff meeting."

"If there were a manager or supervisor who was hired after that training session was given on the Americans with Disabilities Act, what training or education would that manager or supervisor receive on the Americans with Disabilities Act?"

"As far as I know, we had no formal training specifically on the act. All managers were given a copy of our policies and procedures as well as the Employee Handbook and upon promotion they were given just a general orientation to the document that they should be familiar with as managers."

"What was your responsibility in the human relations department for the administration of the Americans with Disabilities Act?"

"I had no specific responsibilities having to do with that act other than to counsel employees and managers within my group if it should come up."

"Were you familiar in 1996 with the provisions of the ADA?"

"Yes, generally."

"What did you understand it to require of an employer such as Connaught at that time?"

"If the employee required an accommodation in order to continue their employment, it was my understanding that the employee could request the accommodation and that the company should comply."

"Did you ever review the technical assistance manual concerning the Americans with Disabilities Act?"

"No."

"Were you ever provided with any manuals or brochures or publications at all concerning the Americans with Disabilities Act?"

"No."

"Was there anyone previously in the human relations department in 1996 who was responsible for ensuring that the rules and regulations of the Americans with Disabilities Act was followed?"

"As a matter of policy, the vice president of human resources I believe was the responsible party for assuring that all laws and regulations were carried out."

"You have been here through the trial so far. In fact you have Multiple Sclerosis?"

"Yes."

"You had Multiple Sclerosis in 1995 and 1996?"

"Yes."

"You were familiar with the symptoms of Multiple Sclerosis?"

"Yes."

"And you yourself have had symptoms, including your hands going numb?"

"Yes."

"Difficulty with fine motor movement?"

"Yes."

"You become easily fatigued?"

"I wouldn't say that, no."

"You won't say that, okay. Obviously you have difficulty walking?"

"Yes."

"You don't know what you are going to experience with your condition from one day to the next, correct?"

"Correct."

"You knew how the effects of those symptoms of Multiple Sclerosis could affect your ability to do your job?"

"Yes."

"In fact in 1996 Connaught accommodated you by allowing you to work at home."

Greco stood up. "Objection, Your Honor, relevance. May I approach?"

"Sustained."

Patrick and Greco approached the bench.

Greco started: "Your Honor, we talked this morning about employees with their own problems. We're talking here about Miss Kirby. Miss Kirby can testify about what she knows about Jane Gagliardo, her condition, what the company has done or not done. I don't want to open the door to come back later on because now she's testifying, everybody gets to testify about their problem."

"Maybe you offered her for a different purpose?" the judge asked.

Patrick said, "She is a very unique situation. Number one, she has the disease, knows about the disease, knows the effects of the disease. Number two, she is a human resources person. She's familiar with the ADA, the responsibilities of ADA, and in fact she's required, as a part of her job, to follow the mandates of ADA."

"You have established that," the judge agreed.

He continued, "Now I'm going to present testimony that she knew what Jane Gagliardo's condition was in 1996, that she knew what problems that she was having, she knew specifically that Jane told her MS was affecting her ability to work. Given all of that she—"

"I don't think he's objecting to any of that."

"I understand that, but the fact that she's working at home shows that she knew an accommodation could be made for someone with MS, and therefore she had even further of an obligation with that knowledge to make sure there was an accommodation. One thing it goes to show and that is she's been identified as the corporate representative.

She works at home. She is not an officer. She is not a supervisor. She has no managerial responsibilities whatsoever. She's sitting here for one purpose and one purpose only."

"Here's the thing. I think it's questionable for the purpose that you stated. I'm not going to go over that again," Judge Kane said. "However, I think it shows bias or potential bias on the part of the witness. He's saying the company accommodated her. She's going to have certain allegiance to the company on the issue about what she's going to testify."

"That's fine, Your Honor, but—" Greco said.

"You accommodated her, you trained her well, you have a lawyer. Not only do you work there—" the judge said.

"It's just that this doesn't open the door for someone to say because she testified that they accommodated for her."

"The next witness can do the same thing if you didn't object."

"I'm—we're not opening the door here," Greco said.

"I wasn't trying to do that. I agree," Patrick said.

"Thank you, Your Honor."

Patrick returned to the lectern. "In 1996 you began working at home, correct?"

"Yes."

"Connaught accommodated your disability?"

"Yes."

"You have loyalty to them because of that, correct?"

"I have a loyalty because of a lot of reasons."

"Would you agree with me that under the laws of the ADA as you understood it in 1995 and 1996, it would have been inappropriate to penalize an employee for missing time from work in order to get medical care?"

"I don't know whether it had to do with the laws that were in effect at that time, but as a matter of policy in the company, we document absence, and if absence becomes a problem, we are within our rights to discipline and penalize an employee on account of their attendance."

"So your understanding back in 1995 and 1996 was that if an employee was absent for medical care or because of an injury, you could note that and discipline them for that?"

"No, not for one occurrence of absence."

"I'm not talking about one occurrence. If there were several occurrences, up to a hundred occurrences for medical care, medical attention or because of an injury or disability, are you saying under company policy you could take that into consideration when appraising or rating an employee?"

"Yes."

"In fact that was done in Jane Gagliardo's performance appraisals, was it not?"

"It was noted in her performance appraisals, yes."

"In the eight plus years that Mrs. Gagliardo was employed by Connaught Laboratories prior to the time that Judith Stout became her supervisor, are you aware of any warning, oral warning, that she received, or written warning?"

"No."

"Did you have a concern at that time that Mrs. Gagliardo's Multiple Sclerosis might be a contributing factor to her performance errors?"

"At that time, no, it didn't enter my mind."

"At some point after Miss Stout became Mrs. Gagliardo's supervisor she came to you with concerns about Jane Gagliardo's performance, correct?"

"Correct."

"Are you aware that Miss Stout knew that Jane Gagliardo had MS, correct?"

"Correct."

"Were you aware in 1996 that Miss Stout requested information from Mrs. Gagliardo concerning Multiple Sclerosis?"

"No, I was not aware of that."

"You were aware that she had provided memory tapes and concentration tapes, videotapes and audiotapes to Mrs. Gagliardo to help her with her memory and concentration."

"Not at that point in time, no."

"When did you learn that?"

"Sometime after Jane's termination."

"Were you ever aware of Miss Stout providing those tapes to anyone else prior to Mrs. Gagliardo's termination?"

"No."

"You said you yourself do not suffer from fatigue, correct?"

"Yeah."

"Are you aware that fatigue is a symptom of Multiple Sclerosis?"

"Yes."

"You were aware of that in 1996?"

"Yes."

"You agree with that today, would you not?"

"Yes."

"Would you also agree that stress aggravates, exacerbates, the symptoms of MS?"

"I'm not sure. I've not read any documentation to that effect, so, no, I don't say that I could agree with that."

"In your experience when you are stressed, does it affect your symptoms of MS?"

"Not directly. I can't say that, no."

"Would you agree with me that immediately after Ms. Stout became Mrs. Gagliardo's supervisor she was putting pressure on Mrs. Gagliardo to improve her performance?"

"I don't know whether I would use the word pressure."

"What word would you choose?"

"She was doing what she should do as a manager. She was keeping in close touch with Jane's performance."

"Were you in the same location as Miss Stout and Mrs. Gagliardo?"

"No."

"So you wouldn't have the ability to observe the interaction on a daily basis between Miss Stout and Mrs. Gagliardo, correct?"

"Right."

"In your experience in the human relations department did you have occasion to have other employees who were being encouraged by supervisors to improve their performance?"

"Objection, Your Honor, testimony about other employees; it's irrelevant," Greco said.

"I'm not intending that. I'm asking a general question. It's not my intention to go into anything specific."

"I'll allow it," the judge ruled.

Patrick repeated the question for Chris Kirby, who agreed that yes, this had happened before and that it could be stressful for an employee.

"You sat in on some of the meetings between Mrs. Gagliardo and Miss Stout, did you not?"

"Yes."

"Which meetings did you sit in on?"

"When she delivered the written caution, when she delivered the probationary letter and at termination."

"What was your purpose in sitting in?"

"It was my role as the human relations manager, employee relations manager, to assure that everything was being handled according to policy and Jane was being treated fairly."

"There came a point in time where you considered that Mrs. Gagliardo's Multiple Sclerosis might be affecting her ability to do her job, wasn't there?"

"Not officially, no."

"I'm not asking you officially, unofficially or otherwise. Am I correct that there did come a point in time when you felt that Mrs. Gagliardo's Multiple Sclerosis was affecting her ability to do her job?"

"Because of my personal knowledge of the symptoms, yes, it did enter my mind."

"It entered your mind that perhaps the difficulties and the mistakes, the problems—you considered the fact that her Multiple Sclerosis might be causing the performance mistakes that she was making, did you not?"

"Yes."

"Did you ever discuss that with Miss Stout?"

"No."

"Did you ever discuss that with anyone at Connaught?"

"No."

"You were aware that Mrs. Gagliardo requested that the military duties be taken away from her, correct?"

"Yes, correct."

"She felt that if the military responsibilities were taken away from her she could do a better job?"

"Yes."

"She felt that it was taking too much of her time?"

"Yes."

"So she was pressured to get her normal duties done within whatever time she had left after the military duties were done, correct?"

"I don't know if she was pressured. I know that was the complete description of her job was to do both. So I'm sure she felt that she had to get both done, yes."

"You previously stated that under the Americans with Disabilities Act an employer is required to provide a reasonable accommodation to an employee, correct?"

"If requested."

"If requested. Reassignment of the military duties would have been a reasonable accommodation, wouldn't it?"

"If it had been requested as an accommodation under the Americas with Disabilities Act, yes, it would have been reasonable."

"Did you understand the law to require Mrs. Gagliardo to say that she wanted the military duties taken away from her as a reasonable accommodation because of her MS?"

"Yes."

"Who told you that?"

"It's just my understanding of how you go about getting a reasonable accommodation. Say 'I have this disability, this particular aspect is affecting my job because of my disability, and I would like it changed.'"

"You knew Mrs. Gagliardo had MS in 1996"

"Yes."

"You yourself have the opinion, the belief, that her Multiple Sclerosis might be affecting her ability to do her job?"

"That was strictly my own thought, yes."

"You knew she asked for a reasonable accommodation. You knew she asked to have the military duties taken away from her?"

"Yes."

"She was stressed because of the amount of time involved in the military and not being able to do her job?"

"Yes."

"You are saying that in 1996 you didn't think that she was asking for a reasonable accommodation because of her MS, putting all that together?"

"I may have thought it, but I can't speculate unless she says it to me, unless she asks me, unless she tells me."

"So you acknowledge that you thought about that in 1996?"

"Yeah."

"Did you discuss that thought with anyone?"

"No."

"Now you stated that you thought it was reasonable, a reasonable accommodation, to have the military duties taken away?"

"I guess so."

"Do you think it's reasonable to delay acting on that request for in excess of six months?"

"Based on my understanding of what goes on in the customer account management department, it's difficult for them to make changes in the workload. It's a very busy department. I believed at the time that they were doing the best that they could to reassign the work duties to find somebody else to fill in."

"My question is, do you think it's reasonable to delay taking those responsibilities away for in excess of six months?"

"Six months, no, that doesn't sound reasonable."

Tullar wrote on a piece of paper, and handed it to Jane. It read: *They just lost.*

"When you sat in on the meetings between Mrs. Gagliardo and Miss Stout when she was given the notice of probation, there was a discussion in those meetings about taking the military responsibilities away, wasn't there?"

"I'm not sure I remember exactly what was discussed at both meetings. At either one of those meetings I'm sure we discussed the military orders."

"You privately met with Mrs. Gagliardo on Connaught property in 1996, did you not?"

"Yes."

"You had a conversation about the mistakes that she was making?"

"Yes."

"During that conversation you asked her if her Multiple Sclerosis was affecting her ability to do her job, didn't you?"

"No, sir, I did not."

"You did not ask her that?"

"No."

"So when she says that, it's not true?"

"No."

"At any time after you had this private thought that her Multiple Sclerosis was affecting her ability to do her work, did you ever take the opportunity to look at her personnel file, specifically her medical records?"

"No."

"Did you ever consider checking with her physician to see if there were any restrictions on her ability to do her job?"

"No, that's not my role."

"Did you ever consider contacting her physician with a copy of the job description and ask her physician whether or not he felt she could perform the job with or without accommodation?"

"No, sir."

"Did you ever do anything after you had those private thoughts about Jane Gagliardo's Multiple Sclerosis affecting her ability to do her job, did you ever do anything to determine whether an accommodation should be made?"

"No, I did not."

"At that time when you had these private thoughts you were in the human relations department, correct?"

"Correct."

"Let's look back at the Employee Handbook, at the paragraph we previously read. 'It is the responsibility of HR to assure that employees are treated fairly and in accordance with all applicable law as an internal policies,' right?"

"Right."

"And the Pennsylvania Human Relations Act?"

"Yes.

"Were you familiar with the Pennsylvania Human Relations Act?"

"Generally speaking, yes."

"It was your responsibility as the human resources manager for the finance department, the administration department, to ensure that Jane Gagliardo, a nine-year employee of Connaught Laboratories, was treated in accordance with the EEOC policy of Connaught and the Americans with Disabilities Act, correct?"

"Yes."

"Yet not once during the period of time when you were the HR representative for Mrs. Gagliardo did you go to anyone and say, 'Jane has Multiple Sclerosis. Jane is having trouble doing her job. I believe it may be related, the difficulties she's having may be related to her Multiple Sclerosis, and maybe we should accommodate her.' You never went to anyone and said that, did you?"

"No, sir, I did not."

"Please look at the termination document you presented to Mrs. Gagliardo. What did you tell her about this agreement?"

"I advised her to take it with her, to read it carefully. I advised her to seek legal counsel to go through this with her, and then we went through it. I showed her that she had 21 days to get it back to us and that if she indicated that she wanted to sign it, she could change her mind after seven days, and I absolutely did not encourage her to sign it during the termination process. That's our procedure."

"You didn't tell her that if she signed it, it would make everyone's life a lot easier?"

"No, sir."

"Are you familiar with the Connaught termination policy?"

"I was at the time."

"Look at the copy of the termination policy that was in effect at the time Mrs. Gagliardo was fired. Would you agree with me, on page 3, that it says:

> Severance pay will be provided and outplacement services offered to all regular employees when the employee is involuntarily terminated due to lack of ability to perform the responsibilities of the position to supervisor's requirements.

Was Mrs. Gagliardo involuntarily terminated due to lack of ability to perform the responsibilities of the position to supervisor's requirements?"

"Yes."

Patrick read out loud the termination release Jane had been given on that fateful day, revealing that she as well as any heir would discharge any charges against the company.

"So you were willing to give Mrs. Gagliardo $14,500 as long as she released you from any other claim?"

"Yes, certainly."

"Let me take you back to that meeting that you had with Mrs. Gagliardo, that private meeting that you had with her. You requested that meeting?"

"I did."

"What was the purpose of that meeting?"

"In my role as her employee relations manager, I wanted to be sure that she understood what was going on, that she felt she was being treated fairly, and I asked her point blank in the meeting, 'Is there anything that we can do to help you through this situation?' Is there anything the company can do to improve the situation for her."

"I have to tell you I am confused. Previously in your testimony you told us that this was a private meeting between you and her. It was not in your capacity as a human resources person. Now you're saying you were meeting with her as the human resources person to discuss this with her. Why is that?"

"When did I say it was a private meeting?"

"Your testimony previously will bear out what you said, but why is it that you wanted to have this meeting with her privately?"

"I just explained that to you."

"By the way, she asked you before that meeting started whether you were tape recording it, didn't she?"

"Yes, she did."

"Why did you not include Judith Stout in that meeting?"

"Because it was between me, as the employee relations manager, and Jane. I didn't want her to feel pressure by having her boss there to answer in any way."

"When you asked her what you could do for her, what Connaught could do for her, what did she say?"

"She didn't know. She said she didn't know why she was making mistakes. She was sorry she was making them. She was trying to do better, but she didn't request anything in particular from us."

"Did you discuss her Multiple Sclerosis?"

"No, I did not."

"As you look back today on the decision that was made in 1996, knowing what you know today, knowing what you have told us today about your private thoughts about her Multiple Sclerosis, your concerns that she may not have been able—or that the Multiple Sclerosis might have affected her ability to do her job and the fact that taking the military away was a reasonable accommodation, do you think you made the right decision in terminating her?"

"I believe I did my job the best way I knew how at the time, and that's all I can say."

"Thank you."

Greco took his turn at the lectern: "Miss Kirby, let's talk for a minute about the private meeting that you had with Mrs. Gagliardo. Did she at that time say anything about her Multiple Sclerosis preventing her from doing her job?"

"No, sir."

"Now you had had these private thoughts because of your condition that maybe it was in fact affecting her."

"Yes."

"But the plaintiff never said at any time that is was. Is that correct?"

"That's correct."

"So even with your private thoughts because of your condition, did you in fact believe on the day that she was terminated that her MS prevented her from doing her job?"

"No."

"At any time in which you were participating in the decision to terminate the plaintiff did anyone on behalf of Connaught say that Mrs. Gagliardo cannot do her job because of her MS?"

"No."

"There was no perception that Mrs. Gagliardo was disabled in 1996 prior to the time she was terminated, was there?"

"No."

"Objection."

"I'm asking the witness—I'm asking for her perception, Your Honor."

The Judge ordered Greco to rephrase his question.

"Did you have any perception that Mrs. Gagliardo was disabled in 1996 prior to the time she was terminated?"

"Objection!"

"Overruled."

"No further questions, Your Honor."

"Miss Kirby, define 'disabled,'" Patrick said, standing behind the plaintiff's table.

"That her disability prevented her from doing her job."

"That's your definition of disability in response to Mr. Greco's question?"

"Yes."

"During this private meeting that you had with Mrs. Gagliardo you carried into the meeting your thought about Mrs. Gagliardo's MS and her ability to do her job. Correct?"

"Yes."

"You knew it was your responsibility, according to the Employee Handbook and according to your prior testimony, to assure that employees were treated fairly in accordance with all applicable laws and internal policies?"

"Yes."

"You knew that Connaught considered its employees to be its most important resource and critical to the achievement of corporate goals and objectives?"

"Yes."

"When Mrs. Gagliardo told you that she didn't know why she was making mistakes, why didn't you ask her the obvious question about Multiple Sclerosis?"

"Putting myself into Jane's position, I would not expect someone to ask me that question. There have been times in my job where I have made mistakes, and if my boss comes to me and asks why have you made this mistake, I would never expect him to say, 'Did you make this mistake because you have Multiple Sclerosis?' I've never had that happen, and people know I have MS."

"I fully appreciate that. However, your situation is unique because like Mrs. Gagliardo, you have MS, right?"

"Yes."

"You know how it affects you?"

"Yes."

"You had thoughts it might be affecting her?"

"It's possible, yes."

"But you never felt as the human resources person to ask her whether or not your private thoughts were correct?"

"I didn't think it was appropriate for me, no."

The atmosphere in the courtroom felt as if an electrical storm had just been unleashed. Jurors were engaged, sitting upright in their chairs, their eyes fastened on Kirby.

"The jurors are primed. Time to call Judy to the stand," Patrick said to Jane and Tullar.

Judy strolled up to the stand as only Judy could. She took the oath to tell the truth. Never once did she look at Jane. She was the face of Connaught, just as Chris had become the face of disability.

Jane felt her spine stiffen and her breath shorten.

Patrick carried the bound deposition manuscript with him to the lectern.

"Would you look at page 235 of your deposition starting at line seven please. You had have an opportunity to read your deposition before it was put in final form, correct?"

"Yes, I did." Stout seemed to wiggle in her chair.

"And you signed your deposition indicating that everything contained in the deposition was transcribed accurately?"

"Yes."

"Would you read line seven please."

"'When you and Chris Kirby discussed Jane's termination, was the fact that Jane had Multiple Sclerosis brought up at all?'"

"And would you read your answer."

"'I don't recall what we said. We may have said, is there anywhere else we could put her, but based on what she told both of us, we felt there was no place in the company, and illness was not a factor.'"

"Would you read the next question please?"

"'What do you mean based on the things she had told you there was no other job for her at Connaught?'"

"And your answer?"

"'If you can't remember what you should be doing; there is no place in the company that you can work. You have to remember what you're doing.'"

"Thank you. I have no other questions." He sat down.

Greco stood. "Miss Stout, what did you mean by that answer to Mr. Reilly when you said: 'Well, if you can't remember what you should be doing, there is no place in the company you can work. You have to remember what you're doing.' What did you mean by that?"

"Each time that Mrs. Gagliardo and I had a discussion about the errors that were made, she repeatedly said to me, 'I don't remember why I made the mistake.' So what I was intending to say was that she could not remember why she made the mistakes. I did not mean to say that she was having a memory problem."

"Did Mrs. Gagliardo ever tell you that she was having a memory problem?"

"No, she did not."

"In fact, with respect to her memory, is the only thing she told you was, 'I can't remember why I made the mistakes,' you discussed with her?"

"That is correct."

Patrick resumed his questioning. He opened the deposition: "Your testimony today is that you did not mean to say that she was having a memory problem during you deposition on May 13, 1998?"

"That is correct."

"Now you were placed under oath at that time, weren't you?"

"Yes."

"You swore to tell the truth at that time?"

"Yes."

"You had a chance after that deposition to take a copy of your deposition transcript and read it, yes?"

"Yes."

"You had a chance to make any corrections at that time to things that were in your deposition transcript, correct?"

"Correct."

"You didn't make any changes to your deposition transcript, did you?"

"No."

"Prior to today you didn't tell me or the court reporter that what you meant to say here is something different than what you actually said?"

"No."

"I have no other questions."

Greco asked: "Mrs. Stout, do you deny that you made that statement in 1998?"

"No, I do not."

"By that statement what did you mean?"

"What I meant was that Mrs. Gagliardo consistently told me that she did not remember why she made the mistakes. She never once told me that she had a memory problem other than she did not remember why she made those particular mistakes on those particular days."

"Now let me ask you, were you nervous at the day that your deposition was taken?"

"Yes, I was."

"No further questions."

Reilly was up to bat. "Were you nervous when you were sitting at your home or wherever you were sitting reading that deposition transcript?"

"No, probably not."

"You stated in response to Mr. Greco's questions that you never once said or Mrs. Gagliardo never once said she had a memory problem."

"Correct."

"Didn't you provide audiotapes to help her with her memory?"

"To enhance her memory."

"To enhance her memory. Thank you."

"Thank you, you may step down," Judge Kane said.

"Plaintiff rests, Your Honor."

At lunch, Patrick told Jane that Judy's arrogance was palpable; it betrayed her own testimony. "She didn't know when to quit."

CHAPTER THIRTY

In for the Kill

———◊———

Back in the courtroom the following Monday, Greco started direct examination of Judy Stout, after the judge reminded Judy that she was still under oath.

Jane wondered, when someone is under oath during a trial, when is the expiration date for telling the truth?

"Good morning, Miss Stout. How long did you know Mrs. Gagliardo?"

"She worked in the same department as I did."

"When did the plaintiff come under your supervision?"

"January 26 of 1996."

"Did there come a time in early 1996 that you became aware of the quality of Mrs. Gagliardo's performance?"

"Yes. I received information from other managers within our group and from the sales force."

"What did you do when you received that information?"

"I researched each of the issues and had a discussion with Mrs. Gagliardo."

Greco directed the attention to the Defendant's Exhibit of handwritten notes made during a meeting on February 27, 1996. Judy said she discussed the errors that had been reported, how Jane had not disputed any of the errors, and how Jane had not indicated she was having problems with her memory. He asked Judy about the military orders special project and repeated Judy's oral and written cautions. Then he had Judy rehash the mistakes Jane had made that led to her termination.

"Do you know whether Mrs. Gagliardo had Multiple Sclerosis?"

"Yes, I did."

"How did you come to learn that she has Multiple Sclerosis?"

"I overheard some of the staff talking in the luncheon indicating that Jane had MS."

"Do you recall when Mrs. Gagliardo first told you she had MS?"

"It would have been sometime in late January."

"What were the circumstances under which you learned she had MS?"

"We were placed in trailers temporarily while a new building was being built, and I had staff that stretched over five trailers, so it was not an easy task for them to get to me, so I would walk around periodically and do a check in and say, 'How are you doing? Do you need anything and so forth?' That particular day I was at Mrs. Gagliardo's work station and I asked her how she was doing, and she proceeded to tell me, she said, 'You know I have MS.' I said, 'Oh, I'm not sure I know much about that disease.'"

"Did she ask you anything after that?"

"She asked me if I would like more information on it, and I said that would be fine."

"Do you know if she sent information to you?"

"I did receive a packet in the mail, yes."

"Did you ever have any other discussion with Mrs. Gagliardo about her Multiple Sclerosis after that?"

"No, I did not."

"Now you say that she sent you information?"

"Yes. It was in an envelope that was in my box. I never opened the envelope."

"Why didn't you open the envelope?"

"Because MS was not an issue in her performance."

"Did she ever, after the time you had that conversation with her in late January 1996, tell you that her Multiple Sclerosis was affecting her ability to do her job?"

"No, she did not."

"Did you ever see Mrs. Gagliardo exhibit any unusual physical symptoms."

"No, I did not."

"Knowing that she had Multiple Sclerosis did you ever feel that perhaps some of the errors she was making were as a result of her MS?"

"No."

"Were you uncomfortable because Mrs. Gagliardo had Multiple Sclerosis?"

"No."

"Why was Mrs. Gagliardo terminated?"

"She was making too many errors."

"Did you regard Mrs. Gagliardo as being disabled because of her MS?"

"No, I did not."

"I have no further questions, Your Honor."

It was Patrick's turn for cross-examination. He had been preparing for this moment for years. A kind of red-hot heat rushed through him as he stepped to the lectern with Judy's deposition in hand. It would barely leave his hand during the course of his questioning. Judy was the antagonist, and the tension was as thick as her narcissism.

"You testified previously that when your deposition was taken on May 13 of 1998, you were nervous, correct?"

"Yes."

"You felt you were under stress?"

"I was nervous, yes."

"That's stress, isn't it?" Patrick glanced at the jurors who were smiling.

"Yes."

"Therefore you were trying to explain that perhaps what you said in your deposition was not what you really meant, correct?"

"What I said is I explained it very poorly in my deposition."

"Are you under stress today?" Patrick's tone was sarcastic.

"I'm under a bit of stress, yes."

"Are you sure you're going to be able to testify without testifying poorly? I'm not saying what you'll—"

One of the jurors chuckled out loud—it was the siren call to go in for the kill.

"I will do my best."

"You'll do your best, okay. So you would admit, would you not, that people who are under stress can make mistakes?"

"That is conceivable, yes."

"It can affect your performance?"

"Yes."

"Mr. Greco asked you some questions about your deposition, and you testified about what you said."

"Yes."

"Prior to becoming Mrs. Gagliardo's supervisor, what did you do at Connaught?"

"I was a paralegal."

"Did you ever have any training on the Americans with Disabilities Act?"

"I'm not sure."

"Did you have any training in the Pennsylvania Human Relations Act?"

"No."

"Do you know if Connaught offered any training to you on the Americans with Disabilities Act prior to the time that Mrs. Gagliardo was terminated?"

"I don't know."

"Prior to being Mrs. Gagliardo's supervisor had you known Jane Gagliardo?"

"Yes."

"Did you first meet her when you began working at Connaught?"

"No."

"You knew her before that?"

"Yes."

"Did you know before you became her supervisor that she had Multiple Sclerosis?"

"Yes."

"Where did you hear it?"

"It would have been somewhere in the cafeteria."

"What was it that you recall hearing?"

"I overheard others speaking that Jane had MS."

Reilly asked Judy about an accident report dated January 12, 1996 before Judy had become Jane's supervisor. He read the report for the jury:

Tonight we had an accident. As everyone is aware, we do not go home when the plant closes early but work our regular hours, until 8 PM. Jane Gagliardo went to her van which is parked in the handicapped section by Building 32. Jane suffers MS.

That accident report was filled out by you?"

"Partially by me, yes."

"And it's signed by you?"

"Yes."

"That was before you were Mrs. Gagliardo's supervisor?"

"Yes."

"And that was in reference to a fall which she had in the parking lot on some ice at Connaught Laboratories, correct?"

"On snow."

"This is a document that you had in your possession January 14, 1996?"

"Yes."

"So you knew at least at that time before you became Jane's supervisor that she had MS?"

"Yes."

"At some point in time you requested information from Mrs. Gagliardo concerning Multiple Sclerosis?"

"No."

"You did not?"

"No, I did not."

"How did it come that information was forwarded to you concerning MS?"

"I was standing at Mrs. Gagliardo's work station. She told me she had MS. I said, 'I don't really know much about that disease.' Mrs. Gagliardo asked me if I wanted information, and I said, 'That would be fine.'"

"And you worked with her on a daily basis at least from January 1996 through May when she was terminated?"

"That is correct."

"You testified on direct examination that you received an envelope from the National Multiple Sclerosis Society, Greater Delaware Valley Chapter, correct?"

"I don't recall exactly who it was from, but I did receive an envelope of information."

"Would you turn to Exhibit 72 please. Is that the document that was received by you?"

"Yes."

"On what date did you receive the information sent by the National Multiple Sclerosis Society of the Greater Philadelphia Valley Chapter? Are you able to read the postmark?"

"April of 1996 it looks like from the postmark."

"Your testimony is that you didn't open it?"

"Correct."

"You didn't open it because you said Multiple Sclerosis was not an issue in her performance?"

"That is correct."

"In 1996, from February to April 1996, what information did you have of your own personal knowledge concerning MS?"

"None."

"You have no medical background, correct?"

"I'm an emergency medical technician."

"As an emergency medical technician did you receive any training or education in MS?"

"No, sir."

"Did you understand what the symptoms of MS were?"

"No."

"Did you know whether or not MS would affect someone in their daily activities?"

"No."

"Then how was it that you could conclude at that time that the MS was not a factor in her performance?"

"I would have assumed if MS was a factor, she would have indicated that to me."

"So you just assumed that because she didn't indicate that it was a factor in her performance, it was not a factor?"

"That's correct."

"Even though when you were discussing with her how things were going to work, she volunteered to you that she had MS?"

"That is correct."

"Would you please look at the items that are inside that envelope please. There are various pamphlets and articles and things there, are there not?"

"Yes."

"Look at the pamphlet called, *What Everyone Should Know About Multiple Sclerosis*, page seven. Please read the symptoms that are described in that pamphlet."

"'They might include eye trouble, paralysis, shaking, bladder and bowel control, staggering, speech problems, weakness or tired feeling, coordination, numbness or dragging.'"

"Now is it your testimony that you never saw any of those symptoms in Jane Gagliardo?"

"That is correct."

"Please look at the pamphlet entitled, *ADA and People with MS*. Would you look through that pamphlet please. Would you agree with me that that pamphlet describes in general terms the Americans with Disabilities Act?"

"Without reading it thoroughly it does appear to."

"You had that document in your possession from April of 1996 until May 1996 at least when Mrs. Gagliardo was terminated?"

"Yes."

"But never looked at it?"

"Correct."

"Looking at the pamphlet, what does the ADA prohibit? Could you read what it says?"

Simply put the ADA prohibits discrimination in employment against otherwise qualified people with disability. Here are some key definitions. Definitions you should know: Disability is a physical or mental impairment that substantially limits one or more major life activities such as walking, seeing, hearing, speaking, learning and working. Qualified is a person who satisfies the primary qualifications for a position and who can perform these central functions of the job with or without reasonable accommodations. Essential functions: Primary job duty, as opposed to marginal duty, that the person must be capable of performing with or without reasonable accommodation. Essential functions may be established by a job analysis and reported in the job description given to all perspective employees.

"Is there also a definition of what a reasonable accommodation is?"
"Yes."
"What does that say?"
She read:

An accommodation is a modification to the work environment or to the way an essential job function is performed. The purpose of the accommodation is to allow an otherwise qualified person to enter or to continue in employment by removing or reducing significant disability related work limitations.

"Again that is the pamphlet that you had in your possession from sometime in April of 1996 until Mrs. Gagliardo was terminated?"
"Yes."
"And never looked at it?"
"Yes."
Patrick asked Judy about the job description of CARs in 1996 and prior job evaluations.
"With respect to the standards of performance, am I correct that Mrs. Gagliardo performed those standards of performance satisfactorily?"
"No."
"What did she not perform satisfactorily?"
"All situations must be handled in a timely fashion, within two days."
"Let me stop you for a moment. Do you recall me asking you in your deposition on May 13 of 1998 whether Mrs. Gagliardo performed that standard of performance appropriately?"
"You must have; I don't recall exactly."

Patrick was granted permission to approach Judy. "I direct your attention to page 151 starting at line six and ending at line 11. Would you read that out loud, please."

"'Under standard of performance for that second duty a) says all situations must be handled in a timely fashion (two days). Did Jane meet that? Answer: As far as I know, yes.'"

"Does that help to refresh your recollection about whether Jane met that standard of performance?"

"Yes."

"Would you look at Plaintiff's Exhibit 17 please. Those are your notes of your meeting with Mrs. Gagliardo on February 27 of 1996, correct?"

"Yes."

"Prior to the time that you had this meeting with Mrs. Gagliardo were you familiar with the disciplinary policy and procedure at Connaught?"

"No, I was not."

"Was there a disciplinary policy and procedure in existence at Connaught Laboratories from 1994 when you became a manager up to February 27 of 1996?"

"Yes."

"And you became a manager I believe in December of 1994, did you not?"

"Yes."

"During that period of time you never reviewed the disciplinary policy?"

"No."

"You didn't receive any training on the disciplinary policy?"

"No."

"Exhibit 2, if you look at it, is this the employee disciplinary policy that was in effect in February of 1996?"

"Yes."

"In fact it was issued in November 19, 1990, is it not?"

"Correct."

"Would you turn to page four, the schedule of discipline for performance related issues. No. 2 deals with verbal counseling. It says:

Informal feedback which is a follow-up or check on progress from previous performance discussions, or is driven by some incident or issue that has affected performance levels.

Am I correct that there were no previous performance discussions that you had with Mrs. Gagliardo?"

"That is correct."

"So this would have been an incident or issue or issues that affected performance levels that led you to have your February 27TH meeting with Mrs. Gagliardo?"

"Correct."

"The first time that's listed on P 17 is with regard to a customer who had requested a history of their account, correct?"

"Yes."

"This was a problem that existed before Mrs. Gagliardo took over the area which was within your supervision?"

"I'm not sure that's correct."

"Did you learn that this issue had been around for a while, that it was one that Mrs. Gagliardo inherited?"

"Yes."

"So she wasn't the first person who was asked for this history?"

"Correct."

"Didn't Mrs. Gagliardo tell you that she had requested that information from the credit and collection group because she didn't know how to get it?"

"I believe what you're saying is correct."

"So she wasn't the only one who was responsible for this error?"

"That is correct."

"Can you tell me again when Mrs. Gagliardo came under your supervision?"

"January 26, 1996."

"Plaintiff's Exhibit 18 is what?"

"A copy of a note within our system where we put all the notes so that we can follow anything that's happened with a customer."

"That's a note dated January 31, 1996?"

"Yes."

"Five days after Mrs. Gagliardo came into your unit, your supervision?"

"Yes."

"That note indicates that this account was trying to get information, trying to get their account straightened out for several months, does it not?"

"Yes."

"And Mrs. Gagliardo only had it for five days?"

The jurors sighed. Judy shifted her suit jacket as if she had bared too much skin.

Patrick continued to question Judy about Jane shipping vaccines to the wrong office on an off date. "We have had some previous testimony, you correct me if I'm wrong, that the procedure under these programs was that if there was an order to go out on a certain date, before it could be released by the CAR, the CAR had to call the doctor or the doctor's office and confirm that the order should go out, correct?"

"That is correct."

"Then there should be some record that that telephone call was made?"

"Yes."

"In this instance there was no record that the telephone call was made?"

"Correct."

"That doesn't mean that the call wasn't made. It just means there was no record of it, correct?"

"Yes."

"This program, the DOC program, was a new program in February of 1996, was it not?"

"Yes."

"In fact, that program wasn't implemented until January 26, 1996?"

"Correct."

"So it was a new program to Mrs. Gagliardo?"

"To everyone, yes."

"To everyone, and you would expect when new responsibilities are given to employees, they are going to make mistakes initially?"

"One would hope not, but it's possible."

"It happens, does it not?"

"I would suppose, yes."

"Miss Stout, did the entire department receive counsel as a result of the problem with this account history?"

"At a staff meeting of the entire department we had a discussion on it, yes."

"Am I correct that Mrs. Gagliardo was not held more accountable for this incident than any other customer account representative?"

"That is not true."

"If you look at your deposition, page 175, line 10 through 12, would you read what it says?"

"'Were you holding her responsible for it more than the other persons involved? Answer: No, we were not.'"

"So when you said in your deposition that you were not holding her any more accountable than any other person, that was not true?"

"I must have misunderstood your question."

"So that's the second time you misunderstood something during your deposition, yes?"

"Yes."

Patrick asked Judy to review her written caution. "Let's go back to the issue of the shipment on February 26, 1996. Would you agree with me that the return would have resulted from the failure perhaps to do a DOC or to call the DOC in order to determine whether or not it should be released?"

"Correct."

"That would have occurred before you met with Mrs. Gagliardo on February 27 of 1996?"

"The shipment would have gone out prior to my discussion with her, yes."

"What occurred after February 27 of 1996 that led you to raise this as an issue in a written caution?"

"I was not made aware of this until March 12, so it was after the time frame of our first discussion."

"But you would agree with me that the act occurred before your discussion of February 27 of 1996?"

"Yes."

"If you look at your second complaint in your written caution against Mrs. Gagliardo, would you agree with me that this act occurred before your discussion with Mrs. Gagliardo on February 27 of 1996?"

"Yes."

"On February 12 of 1996?"

"Yes."

"Would you agree with me that the third matter complained of in your written caution occurred before you had your meeting with Mrs. Gagliardo on February 27 of 1996?"

"Yes."

"Would you agree that the fourth matter that you complained of in your written caution occurred before you spoke with Mrs. Gagliardo on February 27 of 1996?"

"Yes."

"So there is not one new mistake that occurred after February 27 of 1996 that's contained in this written caution, is that correct?"

"That is correct."

"Yet you felt it was appropriate to go to the next step in the disciplinary process and provide a written caution?"

"Yes."

"Did you review the disciplinary policy and procedure before you went to this next step?"

"Yes, I did."

"When did you review that?"

"I would have reviewed it each time before I would have completed each one of these processes."

"Let's take a look at Plaintiff's Exhibit No. 2. No. 3 written caution:

Takes place when progress relative to issues discussed in the annual review process of a verbal counseling session is unsatisfactory. It involves a written plan for improvement, along with specific objectives, and a timeframe of 3 to 6 months for review, feedback and evaluation.

Is that what it says?"

"Yes."

"Could you please tell us what progress relative to issues discussed in the counseling session of February 27, 1996 was unsatisfactory."

"I was made aware of the additional errors that had been made."

"That's it?"

"Yes."

"Let's look at Plaintiff's Exhibit 26 please. Is that the notice of probation that was provided to Mrs. Gagliardo?"

"Yes."

"That notice of probation is only one month and a few days after she was given the written caution, is it not?"

"Yes."

"That notice of probation contains one error?"

"Yes."

"Between March 22 of 1996 and April 29 of 1996 did you caution or warn Mrs. Gagliardo about any new errors?"

"As I was receiving the errors, if I determined that I had some, I was informing Jane that I did have them."

"Do you have any documentation that will show that during that time period you cautioned Mrs. Gagliardo about mistakes that she made?"

"I do not believe I do."

"The substance of this probation letter is that Mrs. Gagliardo took a biologics order agreement, entered it into the system and released product to be sent to the wrong address on the wrong day."

"Yes."

"Am I correct that the customer did receive the product and did accept delivery of the product?"

"I don't indicate that here."

"Did you ever follow-up to determine whether that was the case?"

"I'm sure I did."

"If you look at the third full paragraph of that letter it says the customer was not lost as a result, correct?"

"Correct."

"Would you look at Plaintiff's Exhibit 27 please, a copy of the biologics purchase order agreement that was the subject of your probationary letter. It indicates that the first shipment date was to be on

March 23 of 1996. Would you agree with me that the document was faxed to Mrs. Gagliardo by Mr. Brothen on April 26 of 1996 at 3:17 PM?"

"Yes."

"The day that the first order was to be released?"

"Correct."

"Would you agree with me that Mrs. Gagliardo was under pressure to get this order out?"

"She indicated to me she was under pressure. I do not know that for a fact."

"She told you when you discussed this error with her that she was under pressure to get his order out?"

"Yes."

"You previously testified when you're under pressure, you make mistakes, correct?"

"It's conceivable."

"This is the only mistake that was the subject of the probation letter?"

"That is correct."

"When you issued this probation letter based on one mistake, did you believe that was within the spirit of the discipline policy at Connaught Laboratories?"

"Yes."

"Did you review the discipline policy at Connaught Laboratories when you issued this probation letter?"

"I would have reviewed it prior to the probation letter, yes."

"Would you refer to Plaintiff's Exhibit 2 please and look at page four, the employee discipline policy. Paragraph four says probation:

This step puts the employee on warning that their position is in jeopardy for poor performance. It is the final step prior to termination, and requires improvements to begin immediately. It is a maximum of 3 months; should the problems persist or show no improvement, this timeframe can and should be reduced.

Is that what it says?"

"Yes."

"Other than this one mistake which did not result in losing a customer, what was Mrs. Gagliardo's poor performance from the time that the written caution was issued on March 22 of 1996 until you placed her on probation?"

"This was the error that threw her into the probation period."

"So you understood the policy of Connaught Laboratories to mean poor performance could be defined as one mistake?"

"That is correct."

"Miss Stout, did you ever look through Mrs. Gagliardo's personnel file during the disciplinary process to determine whether or not Mrs. Gagliardo's performance errors were something that were going on for a nine-year period before you became her supervisor?"

"Objection, Your Honor." Greco stood up. "The witness hasn't seen any of those documents. We don't know what that file is. She is unable to answer whether she went through those documents or copies of those documents at this time."

"I will represent that in her deposition I showed her this file," Patrick said. "She identified it as the personnel file."

"I'll allow her to answer if she can," Judge Kane ruled.

"When I had a personnel file on an individual, it would be in my office in a drawer," Judy said. Her voice was stronger as if she was attempting to cover up a perceived weakness. "As I would be adding things to it, I could have been in that file, but to say that I read every single document in that file, I cannot tell you that I did that prior to any of these times, but I would have been adding to that file."

"I believed you testified in your deposition that as compared to other CARs, while Mrs. Gagliardo may have been in the lower half of CARs as far as performing job duties, you wouldn't say she was the worst. Would you agree with that?"

"If that's what I said, then that's what I meant."

The jurors sat back in their seats, a sure sign that Patrick was exposing Judy's indifference. Every time Patrick reached for the deposition transcript, they smiled.

"I'd like you to begin looking at page 165, line 22 and continuing through to page 166, line six. Would you read what it says please."

Judy obliged:

Would you say that during the period of time that you were Jane's supervisor she performed her duties as a CAR as well as, better than or worse than the other CARs or describe it in any other way? Answer: I would have to say that if I placed all the CARs with 1 being my best CAR, 2 being my second best CAR and so forth, Jane would probably be in the latter half, the lower half.

"And the next question and answer please."

"'But not the last? Answer: I don't recall.'"

"So when your deposition was taken two years after Mrs. Gagliardo was fired, you didn't recall whether or not she was your worst worker in terms of performance?

"That is correct."

Patrick steered the questioning to the Equal Employment Opportunity Commission (EEOC) policy.

"I believe that you indicated that the EEOC policy was not considered with respect to Mrs. Gagliardo in your discussion with Chris Kirby, is that correct?"

"Mrs. Gagliardo's issues were based on performance, nothing to do with what was in the EEOC."

"Do you recall me asking you in your deposition whether the EEOC policy was reviewed with respect to Jane Gagliardo, whether during the disciplinary process that she was receiving warning letters when she was put on probation and terminated that you considered the policy? Do you recall being asked that question?"

"I don't recall exactly that question, no."

"Do you recall telling me that the policy was reviewed with Chris Kirby?"

"I don't recall. If that's what I said, then that's what I said."

"Would you read what it says on page 137, starting at line eight and continuing through line 13."

She read:

Did you consider the policy at any time during the process that Jane was receiving warning letters when she was put on probation and actually when she was terminated? Answer: I would have considered that along with Chris Kirby who was my HR representative. Was the policy reviewed with respect to Jane Gagliardo and her Multiple Sclerosis prior to the time she was terminated? Answer: No, it was not.

"Now you indicated in your deposition that you did review the EEOC policy with Chris Kirby, correct?"
"Yes."
"What about the EEOC policy did you review with Chris Kirby?"
"I don't recall specifically. We would have just discussed the policy I'm assuming."
It was clear that at this point, she knew she was caught in her lies and was not even defending her prior statements or suggesting that she was under stress during the deposition.
"Why would you have looked at the policy in determining whether or not to terminate Mrs. Gagliardo?"
"I don't believe we looked to that for the decision to terminate."
"Why would you have looked at the EEOC policy during the process of determining whether or not to terminate Mrs. Gagliardo?"
"I don't recall."
"But you did look at it?"
"I say I did, yes."
"You looked at it during a time when you knew Mrs. Gagliardo had Multiple Sclerosis?"
"Yes."
"Did you know in 1996 whether or not Connaught Laboratories had a policy concerning making reasonable accommodations?"
"I don't recall the dates on the policy, sir."
"Did you know what the policy was in 1996?"
"Yes."
"Would you be surprised to learn when I asked you that question in your deposition, you said you didn't know what the policy was in 1996?"
"I would assume that the policy is based on realistic—"
"No, I asked you a different question. Would you be surprised to learn that when I asked you during your deposition if you knew what the reasonable accommodation policy was, you said you didn't?"

"If that's what I said then, that's what I said." She hung her head then, as if to deny her own defeat. She straightened up, threw her hair back. The deposition was a breathing document.

"The question was:

To your knowledge does Connaught have any policy, official or unofficial, concerning reasonable accommodations? Answer: I'm sure they do. Do you know what it is? Answer: No, I don't.

In 1996 during the time that Mrs. Gagliardo was going through disciplinary process you knew that she had a handicapped parking spot, correct?"

"Yes, I did."

"Did Mrs. Gagliardo ever tell you that if the military duties were taken away from her, she could do a better job?"

"I don't recall her saying that."

"I refer you to page 242 of your deposition beginning at line 15 and continuing through 18. Would you look at that please. What does it say?"

"'And do you know why she no longer wanted responsibility for military collections? Answer: I believe she felt she could do a better job if she did not have military.'"

"So at some point in time Mrs. Gagliardo did tell you she felt she could do a better job if she didn't have military?"

"That was military collections."

"So you agree that the amount of time that she was spending on military work was affecting her ability to do inbound calls?"

"I don't know how I can answer that question."

"You answered it during your deposition. Would you like to see it?"

"Yes."

"I direct your attention to page 243 starting at line five and ending at line 11. What does it say?"

She read:

Did you believe during the period of time that you were Jane's supervisor that the amount of military ordering and collection work that she was doing was affecting her ability to do inbound calls and ordering? Answer: It had an affect on her inbound calls, yes.

"So would you agree then that it did have an affect on her inbound calls today?"

"Yes."

"Would you agree that together with the CDC (Center of Disease Control) responsibility, the military ordering and collections was a special project that took the most time?"

"Without ever comparing the times, I don't know. It's possible."

"Do you recall answering that question in your deposition?"

"I don't recall, Mr. Reilly. It was two years ago. I said it's possible."

"I direct your attention to page 82 starting at line 10 and ending at line 25. Did you say in your deposition that it was fair to say that the military project together with the CDC took the most time of all special projects?"

"Yes."

"You do acknowledge at some point you may have spoken with Miss Kirby about Mrs. Gagliardo's MS?"

"It would have come up in the discussion not as being the topic, just in discussion if there was something else we could do rather than terminate."

"Why would it come up as a topic? Why would her MS come up as a topic during this discussion if it wasn't related to her termination?"

"It had nothing to do with her termination, Mr. Reilly."

"I appreciate that. I know that's your position, but why would it have even come up if it had nothing to do with it?"

"I believe I said I'm not a hundred percent sure that it came up."

"Okay, you think it may have?"

"I'm not sure."

"All right. If it did, why would it have come up?"

"I don't recall."

"You don't recall?"

"I don't recall that it ever came up, and if I don't recall—I'm just not sure if it did."

"The May 29, 1996 termination was based upon one more mistake made by Mrs. Gagliardo, correct?"

"Yes."

"From the time that she received the notice of probation on April 26th, signed for on May 1 of 1996, until May 29, 1996, you fired her for making one more mistake?"

"Yes."

"Would you turn to Plaintiff's Exhibit two please, the termination policy, page four. Paragraph five deals with termination, correct?"

"Yes."

"And it says: 'If all previous steps have failed to correct the situation, termination would ensue,' right?"

"Yes."

"What situation was failed to be corrected?"

"Errors were still being determined and found, the same issues."

"I'm sorry, but you said one error, right?"

"Yes."

"So you are suggesting that that was the situation that was not corrected, the making of one error?"

"I had indicated that in the previous documentation that if any errors were determined after that, that we would move to the next process."

"So if we begin with Plaintiff's Exhibit 17, which is your first meeting with her on February 27 of 1996, you make reference there to three errors. Right?"

"Yes."

"One of those errors was something that Mrs. Gagliardo had inherited that had been a problem for months, correct?"

"That error was an error that, yes, someone else had spoken to that customer. When Mrs. Gagliardo got the request, she was to comply with the request. It made no difference how many people before the customer had spoken with."

"You previously testified that she wasn't held more accountable for that than any other account representative was?"

"That is what I said."

"So we have those three mistakes. Then we move to Plaintiff's Exhibit 25, which is the written caution, and in that written caution you have already acknowledged that there were no new mistakes committed by Mrs. Gagliardo after February 27, 1996, correct?"

"That is correct."

"Then we move to the notice of probation where there is one more mistake made, correct?"

"Yes."

"Then we move to termination where there is one more mistake made, correct?"

"Yes."

"So Mrs. Gagliardo was terminated based on five mistakes that you raised with her, correct?"

"I count nine."

"In that nine you're counting the mistakes that were made prior to February 27 or 1996, correct?"

"I'm counting all of the errors mentioned in these three documents."

"In response to my question you indicated that with respect to the written caution no new mistakes had been committed after February 27 of 1996, correct? Isn't that what you said?"

"Yes."

"Miss Stout, we have heard several instances today where you've told us that what you said at your deposition isn't really what you meant. You said that at least three times now, right?"

"Yes."

"Let me give you one final chance. Is there anything else that appears in your deposition that you said that you didn't mean and want to change?"

The jurors were laughing. Patrick knew that Judy had lost any credibility with them.

"Not that I am aware of."

When Judy left the witness stand, she appeared shaken. The jurors stared at her as she walked down the aisle, as if to usher her out of the courtroom themselves. Some of them were shaking their heads in what appeared to be disgust.

Court resumed the next day, September 25, the last day of testimony. Mr. Greco called Grace Cooper to the stand, a forty-something-year-old executive director of customer services for Connaught.

Cooper's testimony aligned with Judith Stout's, agreeing that Jane was fired for one reason and one reason only—she had made too many mistakes; she wasn't following procedures.

"Did the topic of Mrs. Gagliardo's Multiple Sclerosis come up at any time surrounding the disciplinary process?"

"No, it did not."

"Specifically with respect to terminating her and the discussions you had at that time, what did you say?"

"I said we had given Mrs. Gagliardo every opportunity to improve her performance and she had not; therefore she had to be terminated."

"Did you at any time consider the fact that Mrs. Gagliardo had Multiple Sclerosis when you made the decision to terminate her?"

"No, I didn't."

"But you were aware at the time that she had Multiple Sclerosis?"

"She had Multiple Sclerosis, but there was never an indication that it affected her mentally in any way, and even physically I wasn't sure there was a lot of problems. It wasn't necessarily always the MS. But again mentally there would have been no clue to me that the MS would have been even linked to this performance issue in any way."

"Did Mrs. Gagliardo ever tell you at any time that her MS was affecting her ability to do her work?"

"No, and I was certain she would if that was the case."

"Did you agree with the decision to terminate her?"

"Yes, I did."

"Would that decision have been made even if Mrs. Gagliardo did not have Multiple Sclerosis?"

"Absolutely."

"Why was Mrs. Gagliardo terminated?"

"For severe issues with her performance."

Patrick cross-examined Grace Cooper. He asked her when she learned that Jane had MS and what she knew about MS in 1995 and 1996. She answered that she understood symptoms of MS as including problems with limbs, slurring of speech, and eventual paralysis.

He questioned her about Jane's annual evaluations: "So you in fact had prepared the performance appraisal which is marked P11 for 5-93 to 5-94?"

"Yes."

"You said that her rating was commendable, met expectations?"

"Right."

"If a nine-year employee is starting to have problems in a short period of time during her employment, wouldn't you think it would be incumbent upon you to find out why those errors were being made?"

"Why, how could I find out why?"

"Let me ask it a different way. What did you do to try to find out why Mrs. Gagliardo was making these mistakes?"

"I surrounded her with people she could reach out to if she could figure out why. She had her employee relations manager, Chris Kirby. She had her manager. She had her buddy coach, and she had me. At any point in time she could have stepped forward and told us why, and whatever the why was, we would have worked with her, but all she said was she was bored and she had some focus problems; that's all we heard."

Mr. Greco redirected. He called Chris Kirby to testify again. He asked her again and again if Jane had ever made mention of her MS when she was being terminated, to which Chris said no. He then brought attention to the private meeting Chris and Jane had.

"At that meeting did the topic of Mrs. Gagliardo's MS come up?"

"No, it did not."

"Did you say anything to Mrs. Gagliardo at that meeting regarding her MS?"

"No."

"Did she say anything to you at that meeting regarding her MS?"

"No."

"Now in your participation in her termination was the fact that she had MS any factor whatsoever in that decision?"

"No, it was not."

Patrick cross-examined. "You used those words 'private meeting,' correct?"

"Sure, that's fine."

"With respect to that private meeting that you had with Mrs. Gagliardo you said the issue of MS never came up."

"That's correct."

"You said that you told her that the errors that she was making were serious, and you asked her if she knew why she was making them."

"Yes, that's correct."

"She said she didn't know why?"

"Correct."

"Was anything else discussed?"

"I asked her whether there was anything that we could do to help her to improve her performance."

"Anything else?"

"No, nothing specific that I recall right now."

"Did you cry during that meeting?"

"No."

"So when she said you did, that didn't happen?"

"Correct."

CHAPTER THIRTY-ONE

Closing Arguments

———✺———

"It's time for closing arguments," the judge ruled. "Mr. Reilly."

"This is an important day in Mrs. Gagliardo's life. It's a day when she has presented the dispute between herself and Connaught Laboratories to you as a jury of her peers. She has complete confidence in your ability to review all of the evidence that has been presented, apply the law to the facts of this case and render a verdict in her favor.

"As you have heard throughout the course of this testimony, there is no cure for Multiple Sclerosis, and that's not the issue of the case. But there is a cure for what Mrs. Gagliardo was forced to suffer at the hands of Connaught Laboratories, Inc., and that is damages.

"We all have our jobs to do in this particular case. My job was to prove to you that Mrs. Gagliardo was disabled, that she could do her job, that she failed in part because of her Multiple Sclerosis and that she suffered damages as a result of that, and my job is done.

"After we're finished arguing this to you, Her Honor will instruct you on the law that you are to apply to the facts in this cause, and one of the things that she's going to tell you is that in 1990 Congress enacted a law to protect individuals like Mrs. Gagliardo who suffer from a disability.

"Your job, as a jury of the facts, is to determine what happened here. In essence you are the supreme court of the facts. You will decide, based on the evidence that has been presented to you, what exactly happened, what led to Mrs. Gagliardo's termination.

"You have to determine that from the testimony you heard and the documents that have been admitted into evidence. In determining the credibility of the witnesses, and that's an important duty for you to do because you have heard conflicting stories, you have to determine who's telling the truth, whose side of the story is more believable or whose individual testimony is more believable than someone else.

"You have to determine this by considering whether the individuals who have testified have any bias, prejudice or motive in testifying, whether they stand anything to gain from the outcome of this particular case. You have to consider the demeanor of the witnesses when they testified. Were they nervous? Were they comfortable? Were they honest? Did it seemed rehearsed? You have to use your common sense, your everyday knowledge, the things that you do in your everyday life in evaluating things when you go back into the jury deliberation room and determine what occurred in this case.

"Now I promised you that I was going to show you arrogance, apathy and indifference. I told you we didn't have a perfect case, but I'll be honest with you, I never imagined the arrogance, apathy and indifference that I told you we were going to show was going to be so evident from the witness through Connaught Laboratories.

"Judith Stout is the epitome of arrogance. You saw her testify. You heard her deposition under oath. You heard her tell you on numerous occasions when she was deposed she took an oath. She had an opportunity to read and review her deposition transcript and to make any changes to that transcript that she wanted to. And then you heard her tell you that she didn't really mean what she said during that deposition. You heard her tell you one thing on direct examination, and when confronted on cross examination, she changed her story. She didn't mean what she said in the particular instance.

"While we are on the topic of arrogance, let's talk about the arrogance of Connaught Laboratories, and I'm sorry, I really don't want to bring this up, but ask yourself why is Chris Kirby here as the corporate representative? She's not an officer. She's not an executive. She's not a supervisor. She's not a manager. She's here for one reason and one reason only because they think you're foolish enough to believe that her being here will impress upon you the fact that they are sensitive to the needs of individuals with a disability. Don't let them fool you.

"Chris Kirby testified. She herself has Multiple Sclerosis and knows the effects of the disease, and as I'll point out later throughout my closing, she herself evidenced apathy and indifference. She knew Mrs. Gagliardo had Multiple Sclerosis. She knew it was affecting her ability to do her job, and she never lifted a finger to help her.

"What this case is about is a disability with an individual who is able to do her job, she was not provided an accommodation, she was terminated, and we have showed you what the effect of that is.

"There are two ways that we can show you that Mrs. Gagliardo has a disability. The first is that she has a physical or mental impairment which substantially limits a major life activity or she was regarded by the defendant as having an impairment.

"With regard to the major life activity again you're going to be told that major life activities are concentration and remembering. So in that respect your job is done for you. You're going to be told that she had an impairment and that major life activities do include remembering and concentrating.

"The issue you have to decide is whether she was substantially limited in that major life activity. That means she was significantly restricted as to the manner, duration and condition that she could concentrate and remember as compared to the manner, duration and condition that the average person could concentrate and remember. In direct response to Mr. Greco's questioning Dr. Barbour told you she was substantially limited in her ability to concentrate and remember. The most damaging portion of the testimony that you heard came from Miss Stout herself when she said, 'If she can't concentrate, if she can't remember, there is no job that she can do here at Connaught Laboratories.'

"Jane Gagliardo knew her job well. She received commendable performance appraisals for all of the years that are in question in this case. You heard that she was a resource to other employees who had questions about how to do their job. You heard the other co-employees testify if they had a question, they came to her. She was a mentor. She knew that job.

"Mrs. Gagliardo was expected to do what other CARs had seven or eight hours a day to do in three hours. She was never given a chance to do just the normal job duties and receive the accommodation that she requested.

"Let's talk about discrimination. We're submitting to you that there were two instances in which she was discriminated against because of her disability. She was fired, and she was not given a reasonable accommodation, and let's deal with the reasonable accommodation first.

"Miss Kirby knew Mrs. Gagliardo had Multiple Sclerosis. She knew that she was having performance problems. She privately, her words, considered that the Multiple Sclerosis might be the cause of those performance problems. She knew that Mrs. Gagliardo had requested that the military be taken away from her. She knew that Mrs. Gagliardo had told Miss Stout that she could better do her job if those responsibilities were taken away from her. She knew that it was a reasonable accommodation to take the military duties away from her. But since Mrs. Gagliardo didn't specifically come in and say to her the magic words, 'I have a disability, Multiple Sclerosis, which affects my ability to do my job, I'm asking that you take away the military ordering and collections as a reasonable accommodation to me,' because those words weren't put together like that it's the position of Connaught Laboratories they had no obligation whatsoever to provide reasonable accommodation to her. That simply is not the law.

"That is an example of arrogance, apathy and indifference. They had a legal obligation to engage in the interactive process. Once they knew that Mrs. Gagliardo had a disability, once they knew that she was requesting an accommodation for that disability, they had an obligation to do something. They had an obligation to investigate whether there were other jobs that she could do, whether there were things they could take away from her in order to allow her to do her job, and they failed to do that. That is the first instance of the discrimination.

"With respect to termination all that we need to show you is the fact that they discriminated against her because of her disability is that the disability was a motivating factor. It doesn't have to be the only factor.

"You can infer from the circumstantial evidence and all the other evidence that has been presented in this case, evidence that the disease made Miss Stout uncomfortable, evidence that she asked for information on Multiple Sclerosis early on when she became a supervisor and then stuck it in a drawer, evidence that she provided those videotapes and audiotapes to Mrs. Gagliardo, evidence that Mrs. Gagliardo requested time—lost time from work because of her MS even though she made it up, evidence that there was a private meeting from Miss Kirby, evidence that there was a stress placed upon Jane Gagliardo to get her job done which ultimately they were setting her up to fall, you can infer from all of that that a motivating factor in terminating Mrs. Gagliardo was her disability. They didn't like it. It made them uncomfortable, so they wanted to get rid of her. There is no other legitimate reason offered in this case for her termination.

"A total of five mistakes were responsible for Mrs. Gagliardo being fired, a person who for nine years had worked for the company and didn't have those kinds of mistakes until Miss Stout became her supervisor. Don't let the defendant fool you into believing that she was fired because of a severe problem following procedures because the first time I heard about severe problems following procedures was today when Miss Cooper testified. It's been said out of desperation.

"It doesn't make sense that you would fire a valued employee of nine years who receives letters of commendation from the company president because of five mistakes we have heard about. Clearly we have proven to you that Connaught Laboratories has violated the Americans with Disabilities Act and the Pennsylvania Human Relations Act. The next issue—and we have shown that by a preponderance of the evidence is damages, what has happened as a result of that?

"You heard testimony from Bruce Loch, a certified public accountant, who came in here and testified about the calculations that he had to determine how much income Mrs. Gagliardo has lost since she left Connaught Laboratories.

"The next item of damages is the emotional pain, suffering, inconvenience, loss of enjoyment of life and mental anguish that Mrs. Gagliardo has suffered as a result of this. No one is going to put a number on that for you. No one can or will put a number on that for you. Only you can determine what that's worth.

"I would submit to you that there is no amount of money that you can award to Mrs. Gagliardo that will give that back to her, but unfortunately that's all you can award to her to try to give it back to her. We're asking you to cure that with appropriate damages.

"Mrs. Gagliardo wants nothing from you but total and absolute justice in this case. If you award anything less, if you award partial justice, remember you're also awarding impartial justice.

"We kept our promise to show you that she was disabled, that she could do her job, that she was requesting accommodation, that she was fired and she suffered damages as a result of that. We're asking you now to do your job, find in favor of Mrs. Gagliardo, find that the Americans with Disabilities Act and the Pennsylvania Human Relations Act have been violated in that she was terminated because of her disability and that there was a reasonable accommodation which she requested and was not granted. We're asking you to find that and to award damage on her behalf. Mrs. Gagliardo has complete confidence in your ability to do that and looks forward to hearing from you. Thank you."

"Thank you, Mr. Reilly. Mr. Greco, for the defendant."

Greco swaggered to the lectern: "This is a discrimination case, ladies and gentlemen. From the beginning that's the way it's been described, and that's the way the evidence has been presented. It has nothing to do about the employee being fired for wrongful termination other than discrimination. It's only a discrimination case, and the case is about Mrs. Gagliardo, no one else. She's the plaintiff. She's the person in this case.

"Now Mrs. Gagliardo brings two claims. One of her claims is that defendant Connaught discriminated against her because they didn't give her a reasonable accommodation because of her disability.

"Now in this case the plaintiff claims that she's disabled, and she claims that when she asked to have the military project taken away from her, that was her request for a reasonable accommodation.

"Now Mrs. Gagliardo was having problems. Her performance evaluations as far back as 1993 indicated that she was having problems performing . . . they talk about the letters that were given by Dave Williams, the president of the company. No question, we don't deny them. They were sent, but those letters of commendation has nothing to do with the quality issue. She could do things right, but she did things wrong, and they have the burden of proof to show that she was discriminated against.

"She had the opportunity to contact her employer, and she never did it. She admitted the mistakes. But she says, 'But because you knew

I had Multiple Sclerosis, because you knew I had MS, you were supposed to tell me—Jane, you have MS. Your performance isn't the way it should be; it's got to be your MS.' And she's faulting Connaught for not coming to her and not talking to her, telling her, not calling her doctor. She says we knew she had MS.

"The note that Connaught got in 1995 about her MS, and it's been admitted into evidence by the plaintiff, and we even put it in, too, but it's in there, it's a note from her treating physician Dr. Barbour. Dr. Barbour, in fact, and you'll remember when Dr. Barbour testified, he didn't even remember having sent this note, and no mention of this note appears in Dr. Barbour's note. But it came to Connaught, and the note says—it's on a prescription pad. It says: *Jane Gagliardo is under my care for Multiple Sclerosis*. That's it. Is the severity of it, any limitations substantial or otherwise mentioned here, absolutely not.

"Now Mrs. Gagliardo makes a claim that she was terminated for discriminatory reasons. So we're forgetting the reasonable accommodation now. Now we're talking about termination. Judge Kane is going to tell you, ladies and gentlemen, that in order for Mrs. Gagliardo to prevail on this case she will tell you that the defendant must have acted because of the plaintiff's disability or the disability was a motivating factor.

"Now what does the evidence show? Plaintiff's counsel is right: there is not one Connaught witness who testified—that disability was not a motivating factor, ladies and gentlemen, not a factor, period. Mrs. Gagliardo was terminated because she had made mistakes, mistakes she admitted.

"The employer here is Connaught. Connaught is a healthcare company. Connaught is a vaccine company. They have every right to expect that their employees will do their job and do it well. There is no indication ever that she was terminated because of her MS. Did she ever say that, 'It's the MS. The workload is too much?' No, she never said it, never once, and it's a job that she loved. It's a job that she wanted to hold until the day she retired. She herself told you that she wanted to stay there but she said, 'As long as I was a good employee, I thought I could stay.' Well, she made mistakes. She wasn't a good employee, and that's why she couldn't have stayed. It has nothing to do with discrimination.

"All of the Connaught witnesses testified that the disability was not a motivating factor. And Judge Kane will tell you that where it's not a motivating factor, the plaintiff cannot make out her claim for discrimination.

"So the reasonable accommodation claim is gone. The discrimination claim, there is no evidence, there is not a shred of evidence that Mrs. Gagliardo was terminated because of her MS.

"Now, talking about damages. Judge Kane is going to instruct you that just because she gives an instruction on damages doesn't mean the plaintiff is entitled to damages.

"The question in this case is: was Mrs. Gagliardo disabled? Did she have a disability under the law? Now under the ADA just because a person does things differently doesn't make out a disability. And just because sometimes she has numbness or tingling or sometimes she has trouble focusing, that doesn't make out a disability. But she offered Dr. Barbour to support her claim that she's disabled. If you look at his records, he never found her to be prevented from doing anything. He never prescribed anything for her. He never prescribed any aid to walk or hear or see, never prescribed anything, never imposed any limitations on her. Is that a person who is substantially limited in any life activity? He never found her to have any cognitive dysfunction.

"Then we heard one final thing, and that is that there was a meeting between Chris Kirby and Mrs. Gagliardo. And at that meeting Chris Kirby asked her, 'Jane, is it your MS?' Now no one else was there. No one else was there. And Mrs. Gagliardo said, 'She asked me, and I told her, and from that point forward Connaught really knew.'

"You have taken an oath. You have heard the evidence in this case, and now you're going to retire after you're charged and make your decision. You'll make it based on the evidence and your common sense impressions, your common sense, and you evaluate the evidence in light of your common sense. And you go back in there, and get a jury form, I want you to answer every question, no, no, she was not discriminated against. No, we did not violate her rights under the Americans with Disabilities Act or deny her any reasonable accommodation. Answer no. Make it clear. Mrs. Gagliardo never made it clear, but now what she says is not a perfect case. She wants to hold Connaught because she says we're not perfect.

"It's never been said that Multiple Sclerosis had anything to do with any action the company took against the plaintiff. Thank you very much."

"Thank you, Mr. Greco. Mr. Reilly, I think you have about three minutes."

"Thank you, Your Honor," Patrick said. "What Mr. Greco may have told you is the law or what he expects the judge to say is the law is not the law. Just as what I might say to you or what I might think is the law is not necessarily the law. It's what comes from the bench, the instructions that you receive as to what the law is. It doesn't mean what any perception may be about what a disability is, whether a disability means a person has difficulty walking, a person has difficulty using arms or limbs or breathing or whatever; that's not the disability that you are going to determine in this case. The disability that you will determine whether Mrs. Gagliardo is disabled is under the law of the Americans with Disabilities Act as it will be defined for you, and I would submit to you we have proven that case.

"There doesn't need to be any limitations imposed upon Mrs. Gagliardo by Dr. Barbour. There doesn't need to be a note from Dr. Barbour that says she can or cannot do these things. That's not what the law requires. All Connaught Laboratories has to know is that she has the disability and that's she requested an accommodation, and from that point forward they are required to conduct an investigation. They did not.

"Mr. Greco points out that Dr. Barbour's notes do not indicate that Mrs. Gagliardo said she was having problems with concentration or memory. You also heard Dr. Barbour say he relies on the patient to self report. He only saw her every six months or every year, and just because she didn't complain about it doesn't mean it didn't happen. You have heard plenty of evidence that it did happen.

"Again, finally with respect to what part Mrs. Gagliardo's MS played in their determination to terminate her, keep in mind one thing, Miss Stout admitted to you that during the termination process she and Mrs. Kirby had a conversation about the equal opportunity law. If the MS wasn't a factor, why did they have to consider it? Thank you."

Judge Kane instructed the jury on the law and on the kinds of evidence—direct evidence and circumstantial evidence, and the ADA.

"The claims before you are based on a federal law known as the Americans with Disabilities Act or the ADA and a state law known as the Pennsylvania Human Relations Act, the PHRA. The ADA provides in part that: No covered entity shall discriminate against a qualified individual with a disability because of the disability of such an individual in regard to job application procedures, the hiring, advancement or discharge of employees, employee compensation, job training and other terms, conditions and privileges of employment. The purpose of the Americans with Disabilities Act and the relevant provisions of the PHRA is to provide a clear and comprehensive national policy to eliminate discrimination in the workplace against individuals with disabilities.

"If you return a verdict for plaintiff, then you must award her such money as you believe will fairly and justly compensate the plaintiff for any loss sustained as a direct consequence of the conduct of the defendant. The damages you award must be fair and reasonable, neither inadequate nor excessive.

"In addition to damages for loss of pay, a prevailing party in an ADA action is entitled to damages for emotional pain, suffering, inconvenience, loss of enjoyment of life and mental anguish the plaintiff suffered as a result of the defendant's conduct."

The jurors left to deliberate at 3:17 PM. They returned an hour later.

Jane stood alongside Patrick. She grabbed his hand. She stared at the jurors, who were watching and smiling at her.

"I understand that you have a verdict," Judge Kane said. "Will the foreperson deliver the verdict, please."

The clerk unfolded the form. "Question No. 1. Has plaintiff proven by a preponderance of the evidence that defendant discriminated against her in violation of the Americans with Disabilities Act and the Pennsylvania Human Relations Act by terminating her employment?

"Answer: 'Yes.'"

John, standing behind Jane, placed his hand on her shoulder and squeezed. She felt his strength and relief seep down into her bones.

"No. 2. Has plaintiff proven by a preponderance of the evidence that defendant discriminated against her in violations of the Americans with Disabilities Act and the Pennsylvania Human Relations Act by failing to reasonably accommodate her disability?"

"Answer: 'Yes.'"

"No. 3. What amount of damages, if any, do you award plaintiff to compensate her for the loss of pay, emotional pain, suffering, inconvenience, loss of enjoyment of life and mental anguish that resulted from defendant's violation of the Americans with Disabilities Act and the Pennsylvania Human Relations Act?"

The clerk paused. Her eyes widened. She glanced up at the jurors, then slid her eyes to Jane. She read: "Answer: $2 million."

Jane uttered a sound like someone coming up for air after being underwater too long. Tears flowed. She mouthed a thank you to the jurors and sobbed as she leaned against Pat to steady her. She spun around to embrace John, whose arms seemed to wrap around her body twice.

"Jurors, there is one other matter I need to present for your consideration," Judge Kane said, "regarding punitive damages."

Patrick stood in front of the lectern.

"We are asking you to award punitive damages against Connaught Laboratories. The purpose of punitive damages is to punish someone for the conduct that they have committed and to deter others from committing the same or similar type of conduct." He pounded his fist against the podium.

"We are asking you to punish Connaught Laboratories for what they did, tell them that it's not okay to treat people like they treated Mrs. Gagliardo. I'm asking you to consider punitive damages in this case and award what is fair but send a message to Connaught and others like them."

The jury retired and returned to the court room within a half hour. Once again the clerk read the verdict.

"Do you award punitive damages for defendant's violation of the Americans with Disabilities Act?

"Answer: 'Yes.'"

"Question No. 2. What amount of punitive damages do you award?

"Answer: '$500,000.'"

CHAPTER THIRTY-TWO

Grace

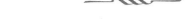

Connaught appealed the decision but the Appellate Court upheld the lower court's ruling on November 22, 2002. Jane donated a portion of her award to the Multiple Sclerosis Society for continued research into the cause and cure of this disease that afflicts so many.

Her parents were both gone by then. They had separated in 1999, after forty-eight years of marriage. Her mother died shortly after.

When her father lay on his death bed, he told Jane and his sons, "If I had known I was going to die, I would have been a better man." At his funeral, five girlfriends showed up to mourn his passing. Even though he had died, Jane couldn't escape him.

From 2003 to 2004 Jane and John worked at their same jobs until Jane was laid off when Bil-Ray closed its doors. She and John set up a college fund for future grandchildren since Johnny, Anthony, and Joseph had all graduated from college by then. Jane's MS went into re-mission in the year that followed, or as someone might say who knows Jane, her MS went into *submission*.

It was a year of dreaming about what their lives would be like now that the lawsuit and appeal were behind them. There was a cushion in the bank, something they had never had before. Their bucket list was short but full: build a home, travel, fly first class at least once in their lives, enjoy their grandchildren, invest some money for whatever med-ical expenses might be incurred as the MS progressed, and celebrate their lives. Early in 2004 John asked Jane to marry him again while kneeling down in their kitchen and presenting her with an engagement ring. Something he couldn't afford to give her over thirty years ago when they were young and pregnant.

After a routine stress test in March, John landed in the hospital for an emergency open heart quadruple-bypass. For the next five months he recuperated at home. He wasn't allowed to return to work until he could pass another stress test.

They bought a one-acre parcel of land in Spring Lake, a small lake community outside East Stroudsburg, and planned to build a simple Cape Cod. On long summer nights they would drive to the property, spread a blanket on the ground, and fantasize late into the evening about how good life would be. There would be an extra garage where John could house classic cars and an in-ground pool in the backyard. The builder promised an early 2006 completion date. On July 4th of that year they hoped to throw the greatest family party they had ever had for their sons and their families, if everything went according to schedule.

Before John might be cleared to return to work, they decided to visit their sons who by then were spread out among Texas, New York and New Jersey. Joseph and his wife Mel had relocated to San Antonio for a teaching position, and their first child was born that summer. They named him John after his grandfather. Jane and John flew down to welcome their first grandchild into the world a week later. On their first evening there Jane found her husband in the nursery, hovered over the baby's crib, crying.

"I've never been happier in all my life. I have never felt this kind of peace," he said to Jane. "I've been given a second chance. I am so grateful to God."

On their way home when their flight was laid over in Atlanta, the airliner announced that it had two first class seats for a seventy-five dollar upgrade. Jane was the first one at the desk. They flew first class for the first and last time in their lives.

After arriving home they repacked their bags and left the next day to travel upstate to Watertown, New York, to Fort Drum to visit their son Johnny and his wife Jenn. Johnny had just returned from a deployment in Afghanistan with the Special Forces a few weeks earlier.

Little did any of them know that Johnny would be redeployed to Afghanistan again two years later. He wouldn't be able to be home when their first child was born.

A week later Jane and John drove to Hoboken to meet their son Anthony and his new wife Laurie for dinner. John told Anthony how good he felt, and that he had one more stress test scheduled for Tuesday that week. It was a warm summer's eve. A breeze blew off the Hudson River, cooling them as they sat outside for dinner.

That Tuesday morning Jane woke up and headed downstairs to brew a pot of coffee as she did every morning. She fetched the morning newspaper and scanned the headlines as she listened to the coffeemaker drip and sputter.

They were scheduled to meet with the builder in the afternoon and walk the property after going for John's follow-up stress test. Outside the kitchen window a hummingbird fluttered its wings so fast they appeared invisible. It reminded her of the cardinal in the bushes she had seen the morning she woke up unable to feel her legs or her arms twenty years earlier. The hummingbird was a good omen, she thought. A small angel.

John's footsteps on the stairs broke her reverie. He was dressed and ready for his appointment at the doctor's office.

"It's a good day, a beautiful day, isn't it?"

"We're happy, aren't we, Babe," he said, "happier than we have ever been?" John paced around the kitchen.

"Happier than we have ever been. Our lives are just beginning," Jane said. She packed an apple and a sandwich for him as he had to fast until the test was over.

They left for the doctor's. While Jane waited for John, she called her friend Toni and they arranged to have dinner together the following night in Stroudsburg at one of her favorite restaurants, *The Willow Tree*. After the test John came into the waiting room and told Jane he had to wait for the results.

"You aren't going to believe this, but Cary gave me the test, you know, that kid who went to school with Joseph. If I pass, they're going to give me my papers so I can return to work."

Fifteen minutes later Cary entered the waiting room with a broad smile on his face.

John stood up like a plaintiff stands up for the pronouncement of a ruling.

"This is the best stress test ever. Your surgery was a great success," he said. "You'll probably live a very long life. You're cleared for work." Then he hugged John.

"You've got to love living in a small town," Jane said, then laughed.

On the way home they dropped the doctor's report off at Yellow Freight, the trucking company he worked for. John would start back next week.

It was a sunny day; the humidity was low for a change. The builder was waiting for them when they arrived at the lake. Together the three of them walked the property, agreeing on how the house would sit and where the pool would go. They marked the trees they wanted to keep. The builder reassured them he would break ground in the next few weeks.

"I know what grace is now," John said that night, before they fell asleep.

The following day, Wednesday, August eighteenth, John complained that his stomach was upset. He downed a couple of antacids but it didn't help much. The builder called and said he had some questions, so they made a quick jaunt to the builder's office to go over more details.

When they arrived home later that afternoon Jane started to make sauce and meat balls for John even though she was going out to dinner. She fixed John's plate.

"I'm not really hungry, Babe. Stomach still isn't right."

"Do you want me to call the doctor?"

"No. The doc said the meds I'm on might upset my stomach until I got used to them."

"Maybe I should cancel my dinner plans and stay home and help you finish painting the upstairs hallway."

"If you stay home I'll get nothing done. All we'll do is talk."

Jane changed her clothes and applied a fresh coat of lipstick.

John walked her to the front door and kissed her good-bye.

"I love you," he said.

Jane met Toni and they caught up with each other's lives. It was around eight o'clock when she started home. Without a doubt she considered herself the luckiest person in the world. Her children were doing well, their new home would be started soon, their first grandchild was healthy. After seven long years, she finally felt at home in her life.

It was only a few minutes after eight when she pulled into the driveway and opened the front door.

"I'm home, Babe," she yelled upstairs. Then she opened the back door to let the dogs out. "I'm home, Babe," she called up the stairs again.

John didn't answer.

She climbed the stairs. With each step gravity magnified. The smell of fresh paint overwhelmed her.

"John, where are you?"

At the top of the stairs she saw John lying on the floor, his feet and legs sticking into the hallway.

"Are you that tired that you have to lay down and take a nap?" She moved toward him.

His body was wedged between the bed and the dresser in their bedroom. The paint roller was still in his hand; his fingers were loose around the handle. He wasn't breathing.

Jane flew downstairs and yanked the cordless phone from its cradle and ran back upstairs, pressing 9-1-1 on the way.

"John, John, open your eyes," she said to him over and over again, until the operator answered.

"I need help. My husband's not responding, he's—" she couldn't say it. She dropped the phone to the floor and knelt next to him.

"Try to keep calm."

"I think my husband has had a stroke," she screamed and cried at once. There was blood and a putrid smell. She saw her tears fall on John's face.

"Is he on his back?" the operator asked.

"No."

"You can't start CPR until he's flat on his back"

Jane struggled to move John to his back, but she couldn't.

"I can't roll him over. I need help. I need help. He's stuck between the bed and the dresser." Jane kept sliding on the plastic tarp that covered the floor.

"A police officer is on his way. I have dispatched an ambulance."

Jane flew back down the stairs to unlock the front door. A police officer was there—he had ridden his bike to her house.

"He's upstairs."

The officer ran up the flight of stairs, flipped John over and started CPR.

Jane called her neighbors. "Something's wrong with John." Within two minutes Pat and Rich Bush were standing next to her.

The ambulance arrived within five minutes. Medics rushed in lugging medical bags, with radios squawking. They insisted that Jane wait in the kitchen while they worked on John.

She watched the shadows of men running up and down the steps. She heard their voices but not their words. The world was surreal.

She didn't know how many minutes or hours had passed when her neighbor came into the kitchen to be with her.

"He's dead, Jane. My God, he's dead."

"But they said he was going to live a long life. Yesterday they said that. I-I was supposed to die first."

Jane started up the stairs again. These same steps that she had climbed for twenty years to wake the kids up, to hide the Christmas presents, to help the boys get ready for proms and then their weddings, to talk to the kids about safe sex, to wake John up to make love to him. No one would ever fit her the way he had.

She lay down next to him on the floor and held him in her arms. His body was warm. She swore she could hear his heart beat.

"I don't want him to be alone," she said to the medics. She prayed that she might flow into him, that just as they had been one in life, they might be one in death.

"Jesus, please bring him back to me—I don't care how sick he is. Please Jesus, bring him back to me. He kept me safe in life; he always kept me safe. Without him I live in my father's world."

Nothing brought him back—not her tears, not her longing, not her prayers.

The coroner came within an hour. Jane refused to let him take John away until John's best friend, Joe Gerry, came to say good-bye. He was so like John—big boned, large in life, more a brother than a friend. Joe knelt over John's body and wept, told him he loved him and would miss him.

They covered John's body with a white sheet and carried him down the stairs. Jane followed, desperately memorizing the contours of his face outlined by the sheet. The flashing lights of the ambulance strobed through the living room causing all motion to appear slow, ghost-like. There was a silence amid the sounds of men, sacred and awful and deep.

One of the medics opened the door for the stretcher. Outside, standing in the road were dozens of friends and neighbors who had seen the ambulance. They gathered to see if John, once the president of the East Stroudsburg Youth Association, who had coached Little League baseball and football to hundreds of children, would be whirled to the hospital only three minutes away. But the men opened the back door of the coroner's car instead and slipped John's body in.

As the coroner's car drove away, Jane gestured to those outside to come into the house and they did, one by one. In stunned sorrow, she collapsed into each one of their arms. Their words paid tribute to what all thought was an unstoppable man; their tears ran like rivers that blessed the dry and airless space, an uncertain geography.

The town ran out of flowers the day of his funeral. To this day, Joseph, Johnny and Anthony believe it was by the grace of God alone that allowed each one of them to see their father one last time only days before he died.

Death—it's one verdict where there is no appeal.

Epilogue

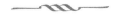

Gagliardo vs. Connaught Laboratories became a landmark case determining that loss of memory and the inability to concentrate are major life activities constituting a disability under the Americans with Disabilities Act. More, damages can be awarded that exceed Federal limitations.

Jane remains in the same house, a place of physical memory, where she and John had lived together and where they had brought up their family. The house on Spring Lake was never built.

In 2008 Jane received state certification to counsel women who are in abusive relationships, to help those who are beaten and battered to stand up for themselves. She volunteered at the Women's Resource Center in East Stroudsburg where women can go to flee abusive relationships, find safety, and restore their lives. That was until she discovered that Connaught, now known as Sanofi-Aventis, monetarily supports the Center. Out of fear that the company would withdraw their funding, Jane no longer volunteers there.

In 2009, five years after John's death, Jane started a local support group called *Weeping Widows* for women to gather and comfort one another, and work to map new lives. She hopes that one day it will become a national network.

To this day people that Jane once worked with at the pharmaceutical company remain distant, out of fear as being seen as collaborating with the enemy. "You are never allowed to step foot again on the campus of Connaught," she was told on the day she was fired.

Justice may have been served in the Gagliardo discrimination case, but clearly it has not been served for all who struggle everyday with a disability to live productive, meaningful lives in the marketplace. But it is a beginning. A message has been sent to corporate America.

"Those with disabilities remind everyone else of their own susceptibility to illness, injury and mortality. Such reminders can beget the impulse to punish those who arise such anxiety," states the Presbyterian Church of the United States of America.

Large corporations such as those of the pharmaceutical industry too often play by their own rules, immune to the law—disposing of employees when they are deemed insignificant. While it may end up costing these corporations in court, have they changed the way they do business? Companies treat their workers as if the employees owe it one hundred fifty percent, as if the company is doing the employees a favor, rather than treating workers for what they are— its very lifeblood.

But when one person stands up for what is right and has the courage to stand against injustice, it begins a transformation, one person at a time. This is Jane's story as she continues to right the wrongs, stand up for the abused and the oppressed, give voice to the voiceless, empower the powerless, and bring visibility to the invisible.

Since the trial, Patrick Reilly has consulted with over seventy-five of Connaught employees for various discrimination and unjust practices cases.

"Every executive at Connaught has your phone number in their desk drawer," one employee confided in Reilly.

On February 23, 2011, the Supreme Court upheld a federal law that closes the courthouse door to lawsuits against the nation's vaccine makers by parents who claim their children suffered severe side effects from the drugs.

According to Justice Antonin Scalia, if the drugmakers could be sued and forced to pay huge claims for devastating injuries, the vaccine industry could be wiped out, reported the McClatchy Tribune News Service.

During that same month, the FDA sent warning letters to Sanofi-Aventis, alleging that the drugmaker submitted 185 crucial "adverse conditions" reports late between January 2009 and March 2010.

So far, the secrets of Swiftwater remain untold.